# BEDSIDE PROCEDURES

Edited by **Gabriel Cismaru**

**Bedside Procedures**
http://dx.doi.org/10.5772/66273
Edited by Gabriel Cismaru

**Contributors**

Gabriel Cismaru, Syed Rahman, Joshua Kuban, Michelle Maneevese, Rahul Sheth, Selim Öncel, Zsolt Bodnár, Cecilia Lazea, Eugenio Martinez Hurtado, Miriam Sánchez Merchante, Javier Ripolles Melchor, Sonia Martin Ventura, Juan Carlos Nuñez-Enriquez, Eduardo Terrones-Vargas, Maribel Ibarra-Sarlat, Lizett Romero-Espinoza, Alejandro Herrera-Landero, Graciela Castañeda-Muciño

**Published by InTech**

Janeza Trdine 9, 51000 Rijeka, Croatia



**Publishing Process Manager** Martina Usljebrka
**Technical Editor** SPi Global
**Cover** InTech Design team

First published January, 2018
Printed in Croatia
Legal deposit, Croatia: National and University Library in Zagreb

Additional hard copies can be obtained from orders@intechopen.com

Bedside Procedures, Edited by Gabriel Cismaru
p. cm.
Print ISBN 978-953-51-3770-2
Online ISBN 978-953-51-3771-9

For EU product safety concerns:
IN TECH d.o.o., Prolaz Marije Krucifikse Kozulić 3, 51000 Rijeka, Croatia,
info@intechopen.com or visit our website at intechopen.com.

# Meet the editor

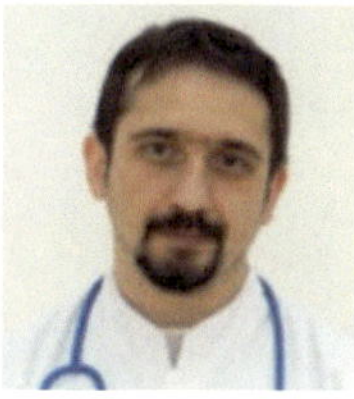

Dr. Cismaru Gabriel received his doctorate in medicine from the "Iuliu Hatieganu" University of Medicine and Pharmacy, Cluj-Napoca, in 2016, and earned his MD degree from the same university in 2005. After completing his residency in cardiology, Dr. Cismaru began his electrophysiology fellowship at the Institut Lorrain du Coeur et des Vaisseaux Louis Mathieu, Nancy, France. In 2011, he started working at the Electrophysiology Laboratory of the Rehabilitation Hospital, Cluj-Napoca. He also works in the Intensive Care Cardiology Unit of the hospital and performs bedside procedures for patients with severe and life-threatening cardiac illnesses and injuries. He is trained to offer close monitoring and support to ensure normal cardiac functions for patients with unstable cardiac conditions. Dr. Cismaru has authored or coauthored peer-reviewed articles and book chapters in the field of general cardiology, arrhythmias, and cardiac pacing.

# Contents

# Preface

Shifting the performance of an invasive procedure from operating room or interventional lab to the ICU has advantages for both the patient and the doctor performing the procedure. *Bedside Procedures* is a guide to interventions that are commonly performed in the intensive care unit, without the need of an operating room. The increased availability of ultrasound guidance increases the success rate of these procedures and decreases the complication rate.

In the following chapters, the authors show that procedures like endotracheal intubation, videolaryngoscopy, pericardial puncture, lumbar puncture, and percutaneous cholecystostomy can be safely performed outside the operating room, at the bed of the patient. Intra-abdominal pressure monitoring should also be used at the bed of the patient to confirm intra-abdominal hypertension and compartment syndrome in patients with pancreatitis, peritonitis, or blunt abdominal trauma.

The first chapter is the Introductory chapter.

The second chapter "Videolaryngoscopy in the Intensive Care Unit" by Eugenio Martínez Hurtado and his team from Madrid demonstrates that videolaryngoscopy becomes and is effective in reducing difficult intubation in ICU patients and remains a basic pillar in survival, evolution, and prognosis in critically ill patients. Compared with direct laryngoscopy, videolaryngoscopy reduces the risk of difficult intubation, decreases the number of Cormack grade 3 or grade 4 views, decreases esophageal intubation, and increases first-attempt success. This chapter of the book ends with illustrations demonstrating the correct airway management and ways to avoid life-threatening complications.

The third chapter "Endotracheal Intubation in Children: Practice Recommendations, Insights, and Future Directions" proposed by the team of professor Maribel Ibara Sarlat from Mexico City demonstrates that endotracheal intubation can be safely performed at the bed of the patient in critically ill children. The chapter describes the rapid sequence intubation procedure, explains how doctors should identify a patient with difficult airway, and illustrates the devices and techniques for the management of difficult airway. Tips and tricks for preparation of intubation equipment, premedication in neonates, ET size selection for neonates, glottic structure identification, and management of deterioration after intubation are described in attractive tables. Pertinent images present the devices used for the management of a child that needs endotracheal intubation.

The fourth chapter "Emergency Pericardiocentesis in Children," written by professor Cecilia Lazea from Cluj-Napoca, describes the technique of echography-guided pericardiocentesis in cardiac tamponade. Images with materials used for emergency techniques emphasize the step-by-step approach to pericardiocentesis. Complications are presented at the end of the chapter, but they are not higher when pericardiocentesis is used as a bedside procedure than in the cath lab or in the operating room.

The fifth chapter "Lumbar Puncture of the Newborn" written by professor Selim Oncel from Izmit, Turkey, starts with a beautiful description of the history of lumbar puncture from ancient Egypt to Heinrich Quincke. The author then presents the indications and contraindications of the technique along with the possible complications and how to interpret the cerebrospinal fluid findings. The substantial part of the chapter consists in the procedure itself, with preparation of the materials, positioning of the newborn, how to take landmarks for the puncture, and how to successfully introduce the needle and aspirate cerebrospinal fluid. The artwork of professor Oncel speaks louder than words, and the reader of this chapter will discover a real artist in medical painting.

The sixth chapter "Percutaneous Cholecystostomy" by Michelle Maneevese and her team from Houston, United States, also starts with a historical perspective and then continues with the indications and contraindications of the technique. Percutaneous cholecystostomy quickly decompresses the gallbladder to prevent gallbladder rupture and resultant peritonitis. When performed at the bed of the patient, it can be guided by echography. Both the transhepatic and transperitoneal approaches are described as well as the Seldinger technique and the trocar technique for catheter placement inside the bladder. Fluoroscopic, ultrasonographic, and tomographic images accompany the specific details of the technique.

The seventh chapter "Intra-abdominal Pressure Monitoring" by doctor Zsolt Bodnar from Letterkenny, Ireland, describes the advantages and disadvantages of the different techniques for monitoring of the intra-abdominal pressure. It is the only possible way of establishing the diagnosis of abdominal compartment syndrome and is based on the measurement of the intra-abdominal pressure through the bladder. The author proposes the continuous intra-abdominal pressure monitoring, describes the method and compares it with the intermittent method, and validates it as a new monitoring technique.

All the chapters of the book are clinically orientated providing explanations and illustrations for invasive procedures. The information is accessible with a minimal theoretical background, but some bedside procedures may require additional training and experience. Therefore, practical recommendations are given in the book, with figures on the techniques performed in critically ill patients.

It will serve the experienced doctor who has not performed a procedure for a long time as well as the young doctors needing a practical assistance when facing a new patient.

**Cismaru Gabriel, MD, PhD**
5th Department of Internal Medicine, Cardiology Rehabilitation,
"Iuliu Hatieganu" University of Medicine and Pharmacy,
Cluj-Napoca, Romania

Chapter 1

# Introductory Chapter: Bedside Procedures in Critical Care Unit

Cismaru Gabriel

Additional information is available at the end of the chapter

http://dx.doi.org/10.5772/intechopen.73068

## 1. Introduction

The number of procedures performed in an operating room (OR) or interventional radiology (IR) is high; therefore, the performance of bedside procedures may decongest those services and be more rapidly performed by the team that is closest to the patient. It was also demonstrated that it can prevent serious adverse effects related to the transportation of patients to OR or IR. The price for radiology performed procedures is also higher compared to those performed at the bed of the patient as there are specific charges for special radiological equipment, radiologist's time and procedural space [1].

Some of the procedures performed at the bed of the patient may need ultrasound guidance. Ultrasound should be available in the ICU department and portable devices can guide paracentesis, thoracocentesis, pericardial puncture, abscess drainage, insertion of venous central line, or insertion of an arterial line. In the new years, hand-held ultrasound machines made the procedures even more easy to perform as it can be used for the guidance of vascular access or fluid removal from the pericardium, pleura, abdomen, cystostomy, etc. The placement of inferior vena cava filters is performed in patients with deep vein thrombosis and contraindication to anticoagulants or recurrent thromboembolism after correct anticoagulation. Filters can be implanted at the bed of the patient using intravascular echography, available as rotational or sectorial ultrasound. Transesophageal echocardiography can also be used at the bed of the patient to guide implantation of chemotherapy chambers or chambers for continuous high doses of diuretics [2].

Many procedures utilize special available kits for central venous catheter placement, arterial line placement, pericardiocentesis (**Figure 1**), pulmonary artery catheterization, percutaneous tracheostomy, temporary pacemaker insertion (**Figure 2**), port-a-cath (**Figure 3**) lumbar puncture or suprapubic cystostomy. These kits include drapes, gloves, caps, gowns and masks for

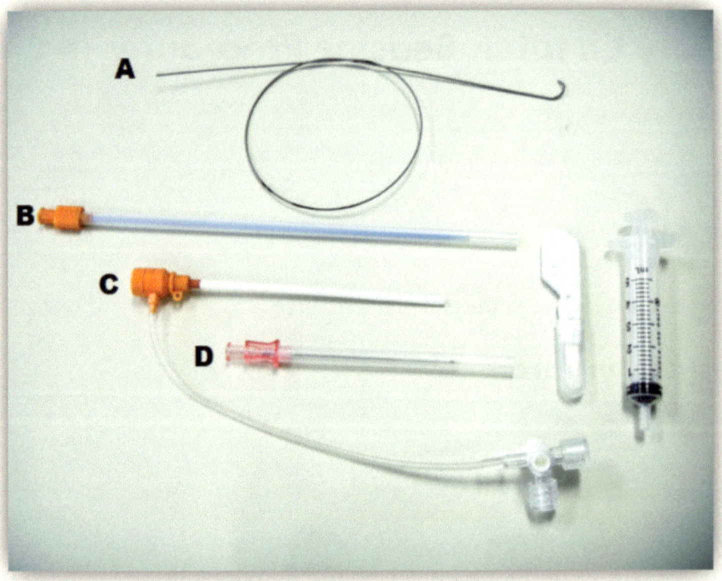


**Figure 1.** Pericardiocentesis kit: (A) atraumatic metallic guidewire that enters inside the pericardium after the puncture with the needle; (B) dilator—is stiff, made of plastic and dilates the orifice made by the needle; it permits the introduction of the aspiration catheter; (C) aspiration catheter; and (D) needle.

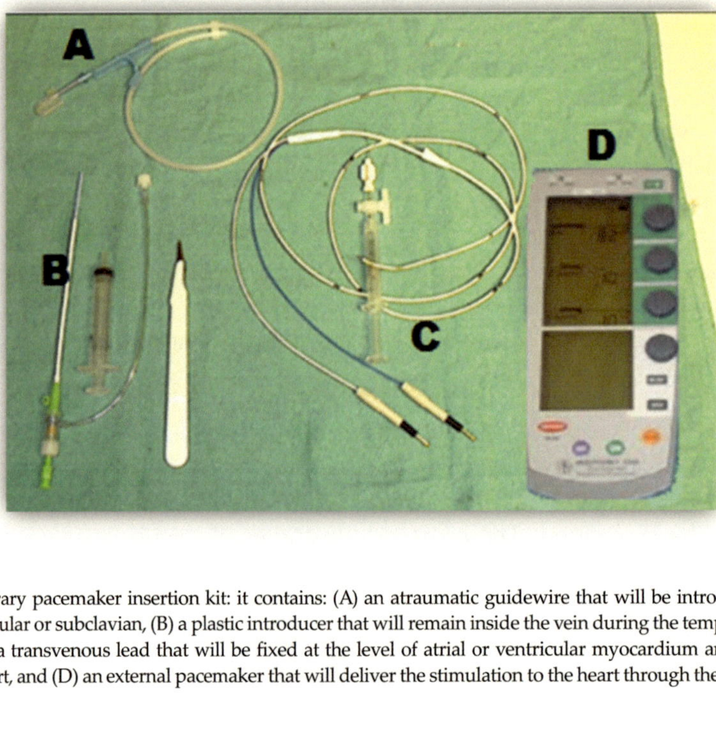


**Figure 2.** Temporary pacemaker insertion kit: it contains: (A) an atraumatic guidewire that will be introduced in a central vein: femoral, jugular or subclavian, (B) a plastic introducer that will remain inside the vein during the temporary stimulation of the heart, (C) a transvenous lead that will be fixed at the level of atrial or ventricular myocardium and will be used to stimulate the heart, and (D) an external pacemaker that will deliver the stimulation to the heart through the transvenous lead.

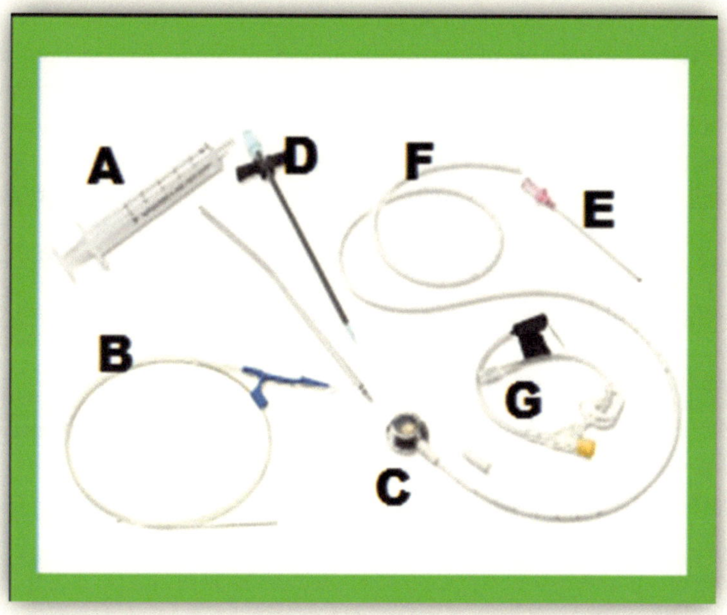


**Figure 3.** Port a cath Implantable Venous Access System kit. It can be used for chemotherapy administration, high doses of diuretics in terminal heart failure patients, parenteral nutrition, and blood sampling. (A) Syringe, (B) atraumatic metallic catheter that will be introduced through the cephalic, jugular or subclavian vein, (C) the chamber for therapy injection, (D) dilator used to access the central vein, (E) needle for venous puncture, (F) polyethylene catheter tubing that will be inserted at the junction between the right atrium and superior vena cava, and (G) 90-degree winged infusion set.

the doctor, betadine, needles, catheters, blades, syringes, drainage catheters, bags, tubes, lidocaine with and without adrenaline, for the procedure itself. The kit provides maximal barrier precautions and also lowers the rate of iatrogenic infection.

## 2. How to perform bedside procedures?

Before deciding to perform a procedure at the bedside of the patient in ICU, we should limit visitors to enter in the immediate surrounding of the patient or even in the entire unit during the performance of the procedure. This ensures a sterile field and also provides measures of privacy. On the other hand, we should separate the procedure and the patient from the rest of the ICU to minimize distractions and disruptions. This can be done by curtains or temporary partitions or by changing the room of the performance. Nurses should be present during the procedure, and they should be familiar with the technique of the procedure. Most of the time adequate sedation is necessary with midazolam, propofol and pethidine. Doses for analgesia and sedation should be prescribed by the doctor, but the volume of the vial and dilution should be known by the nurse. Prior to assisting in a new procedure, nurses, residents, students and other staff members should receive adequate training with a prior period of observation when there is no anterior experience [3].

For the safety of the procedure, adequate preparation is mandatory, with prior sedation, intravenous access, initial preparation of the kit and suitable monitoring. Specific sites for venous access are preferred in the function of the bedside procedure being performed. Advanced airway equipment should be available, especially when the bedside procedure is performed in an unstable patient. Whenever possible, informed consent should be obtained from the patient before the beginning of the procedure, and in case of unstable patients, consent should be obtained from a family member or tutor of the patient. All the staff members should be aware of the nosocomial infection risk. This risk can be reduced by proper hand hygiene, the use of antiseptic skin agents, selecting a good puncture site, and the use of sterile drapes for an aseptic technique [4].

Proper hand hygiene, appropriate site selection, use of appropriate skin preparation agents, and an aseptic technique with a full body drape during device insertion have been shown to reduce the rate of nosocomial device-related infections.

In urban non-academic, rural and community hospitals, intensivists are more likely to perform bedside procedures as compared to their urban academic counterparts. This is likely because of a lack in interventional radiology departments and performance of the procedure at the bed of the patient may be particularly important [5].

We are of the strong belief that hospitalization costs can be reduced by doing the procedures at the bedside of the patient rather than referring them to the surgery department or interventional radiology.

## Author details

Cismaru Gabriel

Address all correspondence to: gabi_cismaru@yahoo.com

5th Department of Internal Medicine, Cardiology Rehabilitation, Iuliu Hatieganu University of Medicine and Pharmacy, Cluj-Napoca, Romania

## References

[1] Barsuk JH, Cohen ER, Feinglass J, et al. Clinical outcomes after bedside and interventional radiology paracentesis procedures. The American Journal of Medicine. 2013;**126**:349-356

[2] Brown SM, Kasal J. Bedside ultrasound in the intensive care unit: Where is the evidence? Seminars in Respiratory and Critical Care Medicine. 2015 Dec;**36**(6):878-889

[3] Thakkar R, Wright SM, Alguire P, et al. Procedures performed by hospitalist and non-hospitalist general internists. Journal of General Internal Medicine. 2010;**25**:448-452

[4] Heisler M. Hospitalists and intensivists: Partners in caring for the critically ill—The time has come. Journal of Hospital Medicine. 2010;**5**:1-3

[5] Wigton RS, Alguire P. The declining number and variety of procedures done by general internists: A resurvey of members of the American College of Physicians. Annals of Internal Medicine. 2007;**146**:355-360

Chapter 2

# Videolaryngoscopy in the Intensive Care Unit: We could Improve ICU Patients Safety

Eugenio Martínez Hurtado,
Miriam Sánchez Merchante, Sonia Martín Ventura,
María Luisa Mariscal Flores and
Javier Ripollés Melchor

Additional information is available at the end of the chapter

http://dx.doi.org/10.5772/intechopen.72658

**Abstract**

Tracheal intubation is one of the most common and dangerous procedures in the intensive care units (ICU), and is usually done in more difficult conditions than in the operating room. Intubation failure can occur unexpectedly, and is the second most common event reflected in the ICU in the NAP4. Complications associated with airways were more likely to occur in ICU than in the operating room (severe hypoxemia, arrhythmia, hypotension, cardiovascular collapse, etc.), and generates more frequent damage to the patient. The theoretical benefits of videolaryngoscopes, as proper and correct use, offer the potential to reduce the difficulty of intubation in the ICU. In recent years, the role of videolaryngoscopes in ICU has been the subject of debate. Numerous studies have shown increased morbidity when performing multiple attempts at tracheal intubation. Videolaryngoscopes allow a view of the entrance of glottis independent of the line of sight, and have also been shown to improve glottis and intubation success rates in emergency and emergency services, in the prehospital setting, and specifically in patients with known predictors of difficult airway (DA).

**Keywords:** tracheal intubation, NAP4, complications, videolaryngoscopes, difficult airway, airway management, laryngoscopy, critical patient

## 1. Introduction

Airway management (AM) in intensive care units (ICU) is a common practice that is usually performed in more complicated conditions than in the operating room, where it is performed on a scheduled basis. The fundamental difference is that these patients are frequently in a situation of

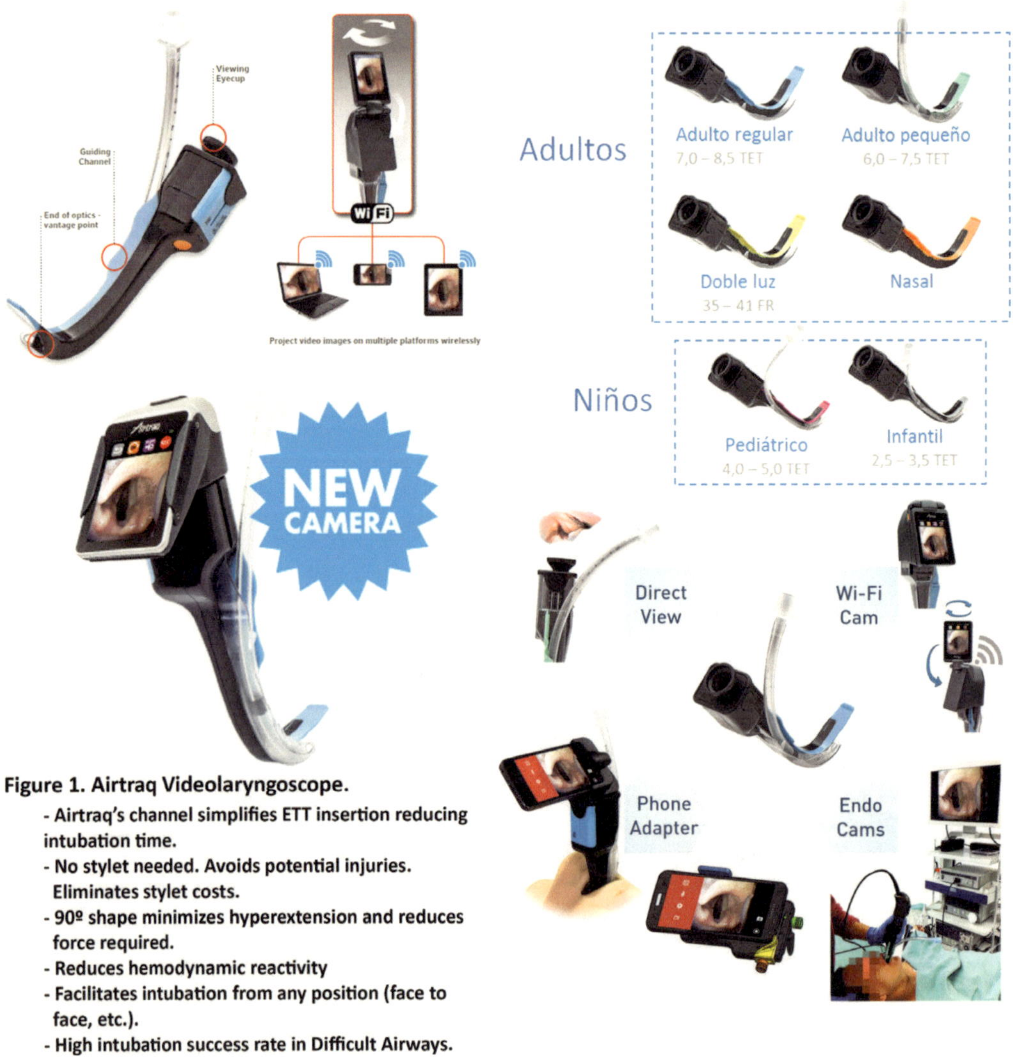
Viewing Eyecup
Guiding Channel
End of optics - vantage point
Wi Fi
Project video images on multiple platforms wirelessly
Adultos
Adulto regular
7,0 – 8,5 TET
Adulto pequeño
6,0 – 7,5 TET
Doble luz
35 – 41 FR
Nasal
Niños
Pediátrico
4,0 – 5,0 TET
Infantil
2,5 – 3,5 TET
NEW CAMERA
Direct View
Wi-Fi Cam
Phone Adapter
Endo Cams
Figure 1. Airtraq Videolaryngoscope.
- Airtraq's channel simplifies ETT insertion reducing intubation time.
- No stylet needed. Avoids potential injuries. Eliminates stylet costs.
- 90º shape minimizes hyperextension and reduces force required.
- Reduces hemodynamic reactivity
- Facilitates intubation from any position (face to face, etc.).
- High intubation success rate in Difficult Airways.

**Figure 1.** Airtraq videolaryngoscope.

hypoxemia and cardiovascular collapse, so in many situations, the airway management in these clinical conditions is often complicated, if not emergency. Therefore, it is usually considered that these patients present, at the beginning, a possible difficult airway (DA).

Although failure to manage AM sometimes occurs unexpectedly, it is known to be the second most common event reflected in NAP4 in the ICU [1]. So, all patients admitted in the ICU should be considered at risk.

The airway approach in this environment has gained interest in recent years, especially after NAP4, in which airway complications were found to be more likely to occur in the ICU than in the operating room (severe hypoxemia, in addition to arrhythmias, hypotension, and cardiovascular collapse), and more frequently caused harm to the patient. This study specifically mentioned the theoretical benefit of videolaryngoscopes (VL), since their proper and correct use would offer the potential to reduce the difficulty of intubation in the ICU (**Figure 1**).

Other important conclusions drawn from the NAP4 were the scarce airway assessment performed in the critical units and did not allow us to anticipate a DA, resulting in poor planning. It was also observed that, in the context of an unexpected DA, the limited ability to modify the established plan may lead to a failure to resolve the situation.

The utility of videolaryngoscopy in anesthesia is widely recognized and endorsements advocating its use have been incorporated in the UK and American Difficult Airway Society guidelines [2, 3].

## 2. Epidemiology

The degree of difficulty with face mask ventilation (FMV) and intubation with direct laryngoscopy (DL) is very variable according to the studies and although the degree of difficulty for intubation does not have to correspond to the difficulty for ventilation with facial masks, if they occur together in the same patient, the consequences can be catastrophic [4].

Traditionally, the difficulty for laryngoscopy vision is difficult to intubate [5, 6].

In general, the incidence of Cormack-Lehane grades 3/4 and 4/4 ranges from 1 to 10%, and 2–8%, respectively. These figures are up to 7.9% in pregnant women requiring general anesthesia, with 2% of cases being *"very difficult intubation"*, an incidence similar to difficult orotracheal intubation (OTI) in urgent non-obstetric surgical patients.

Finally, the catastrophic situation of *"can't-intubate-can't-oxygenate"* (CICO) can occur with an incidence of 1–3 per 10,000 patients to 1 per 50,000 patients according to the authors.

All these figures vary between studies, mainly because there is no unanimity in the definitions or terms related to AM.

Within the specific context of an ICU, the incidence of DA rises to 10–20% [7–12].

Facial mask ventilation (FMV) is a fundamental element of the AM that would ensure patient oxygenation between the different intubation attempts. It has been classically described an incidence of difficulty FMV of 0.08% [5].

In 2004, a scale of 4 degrees of difficulty FMV was established, assigning a score of 0–4 according to the difficulty found [13], which was later used in a study of 22,660 patients [14], Finding a degree of difficulty of:

- Grade 1: easy FMV (77.4%).
- Grade 2: easy FMV with an oral cannula or other adjuvants (21.1%).
- Grade 3: difficult FMV (inadequate, unstable or requiring two operators) (1.4%).

- Grade 4: inability FMV (0.16%).
- Grade 3 or 4 + difficult intubation: 0.37%.

In order to increase statistical power in some variables of the previous study, in 2009, a new study was carried out, collecting more than 50,000 patients [15]. It was recognized that the incidence of impossible FMV, defined as "*the inability to ventilate with facial masks despite the use of facilitating devices and 2-hand ventilation*", was found to be around 0.15%.

## 3. Particularities of airway management in the critical patient

Critical patient intubation is often performed in ICU, but can also be performed in locations away from the operating room, where working conditions and available materials are often inadequate. The difficulty rate of orotracheal intubation in emergency situations is 3 times higher than the programmed procedure, with a reported incidence of 10–20% failure at the first-attempt [7], with a complication rate 50 times higher than those found during anesthesia [1].

The AM of the critically ill patient may be complicated by the anatomical characteristics involving the visualization of glottis opening, or the difficult passage of the tracheal tube through the vocal cords, or by the clinical situation itself, which may contribute to the cardiovascular collapse. Among these causes of physiologic DA are hypoxemia, hypotension, severe metabolic acidosis, and right ventricular failure [16]. In fact, approximately 20% of patients in the ICU will experience critical hypoxemia, which, in the worst case, leads to death. Other common complications are esophageal intubation, aspiration, and selective bronchial intubation, among others.

DA is defined as "*that clinical situation in which an experienced anesthesiologist present difficulties with ventilation with a face mask, difficulty with OTI, or both*". Likewise, difficult intubation can be defined as "*the need for 3 or more attempts for OTI, or more than 10 minutes to achieve it*" [2].

However, despite handling the DA forced to take decisions and perform actions quickly and effectively, the truth is that there is no unanimity in the definitions or terms related to AM, because "the DA not exists, in reality, but is a complex interaction between the patient, the anesthetist, the available equipment and other circumstances" [17].

Until a few years ago, the available systems of evaluation have had in little consideration factors not related to the patient. Some factors that complicate and diminish the safety of the management of the AM such as:

- Experience.
- Pressure of time-urgency.
- Availability of suitable equipment.
- Location.
- Human factors.

However, it is currently considered *"management of context-sensitive airway"*, where a gaseous exchange is more valued than the tracheal intubation itself [18], which consists of four ventilation and oxygenation methods:

1. Facial mask.
2. Supraglottic or extraglottic devices.
3. Endotracheal tube.
4. Surgical AM.

The use of any of these methods depends not only on the devices but also on the situation facing the professional. In this management of context-sensitive MA, maintenance of the patient's gauche exchange is the priority and should not be *"device dependent"*. Thus, careful evaluation of the *"context"* interpretation is essential for the safe practice of MA management.

The concept *"context-sensitive AM"* acquires special relevance in critically ill patients, and there are several causes that make it difficult to manage their AM:

1. Non-patient dependent:
    - Who manages airway?
    - Where is the patient?
    - What equipment and medication are available?
    - Who helps?
2. Dependent patient:
    - Predictive tests of AD.
    - Pathology of the patient (hemorrhage, edema, trauma, increased secretions, etc.).

## 4. Complications of intubation in the critical patient

The primary indication for OTI in ICU is the acute respiratory failure. Weakness and fatigue of respiratory muscles (ventilatory failure) and disruption of gas exchange (respiratory failure) are common, and the risk of hypoxemia and cardiovascular shock during the OTI process is high, ranging from 15 to 50%.

Critical patient intubation presents life-threatening complications in more than one-third of cases [19]. The most common are respiratory and hemodynamic alterations [20]. The main adverse event associated with the technique is hypoxemia with a dramatic decrease in peripheral oxygen saturation (SapO2) despite adequate preoxygenation. In almost half of the cases, the indication for tracheal intubation is due to an acute respiratory failure with a previous SapO2 of less than 90% that supports the appearance of severe hypoxemia.

The second complication due to its frequency is hemodynamic alteration with hypotension after intubation, associated or not with desaturation. Mort reported 60 cardiac arrests during 3035 intubations outside the operating room (incidence of 2%) [21]. About 83% of these patients experienced severe hypoxemia (SatpO2 < 70%). The choice of the drug suitable for anesthetic induction is very important to minimize hypotension in the critical.

Other complications described in the literature are esophageal intubation and pulmonary aspiration. The former increases the risk of cardiac arrest by 15 times.

NAP4 reported that ICU, far from representing a safe place to operate the airway, were a place of potential danger. Airway-related complications were more likely to occur in the ICU than in the operating room, and more often resulted in harm to the patient. Thus, the rate of airway complications that appeared in the ICU was more than 50 times higher than those found during anesthesia, and 61% of the ICU patients reported on NAP4 suffered neurological damage or death, compared to 14% during the anesthetic procedure and 33% in the emergency department. Although most of the potentially fatal airway events in the ICU were due to especially tracheal tube displacement or tracheostomy (especially in obese patients), difficulties were also identified associated with esophageal intubation, rapid sequence intubation, and failure techniques of the rescue of the airways [1].

There are four factors that are independently associated with a serious complication during the procedure:

1. Age is a factor that cannot be modified and is accompanied by a worse response of the organism to any aggression.
2. Second, there are two factors depending on the patient's previous physiological status, the presence of hypotension, and/or hypoxemia conditions an increased risk of complications. In some cases, these factors can be modified by optimizing blood pressure and oxygenation.
3. The presence of secretions in the oropharyngeal cavity hinders laryngoscopic vision and has been associated with an increase in the rate of failure of tracheal intubation.
4. Lastly, the need for more than one attempt for intubation increases the risk of complications. A number greater than two attempts increases the risk of hypoxemia, bradycardia, aspiration of gastric contents, and cardiac arrest exponentially [21].

The presence of two clinicians reduces the risk of complications.

## 5. Approach of the airway management in the critical patient

The aims of the AM, understood as the accomplishment of maneuvers and the use of devices that allow adequate and safe ventilation to patients who need it, is to guarantee the oxygenation in a situation of potential vital risk for that patient.

The optimal AM and ventilation of critical patients remain a basic pillar in survival, evolution, and prognosis, with OTI being the gold standard in these situations.

Most patients requiring tracheal intubation and mechanical ventilation in the ICU are, in contrast to those requiring these procedures in an operating room, patients with a circulatory and/or respiratory compromise. Therefore, the intubation procedure should be non-aggressive and atraumatic.

The cardiorespiratory instability usually presented by the seriously ill patient (with reduced functional residual capacity and safe apnea time), together with the urgent nature of the situation, the low predictability of the possible scenarios, jointly with the fact that it is often not possible ensure adequate gastric emptying, determine that the intubation of critical airway is a high-risk procedure. For this reason, all critical patients should be initially managed as potential AD.

The results of the NAP4 audit are parallel to other studies that consider that multiple attempts at intubation in the critical patient result in a high incidence of adverse events [22]. In order to limit the number of attempts to two and to ensure success, interventions such as an adequate patient position and the existence, at the bedside, of correct material equipment and experienced personnel are necessary.

The assessment of the airway in the critical patient may be complex, but adequate planning should be part of the daily approach to the airway. This assessment must include the factors that predict a DA that we routinely use in the anesthesia consultation. The patient's position, the additional help present, and the available material must be evaluated prior to anesthetic induction. In addition, the physiological characteristics of the subject such as the full stomach and situations that favor desaturation (obesity and pulmonary shunt) should be considered.

The oxygenation of patients before and during intubation is of paramount importance [23]. Premaneuver denitrogenate has been shown to be useful as oxygenation with nasal goggles during apnea. The administration of high concentrations of oxygen through high-flow nasal glasses (HFNG) seems to offer advantages over the classic preoxygenation models. It provides some degree of positive pressure even during laryngoscopy without requiring patient collaboration [24].

Historically, direct laryngoscopy has been the most commonly used method for intubation in critically ill patients. Alternatives such as luminous stylet, supraglottic device, and flexible fibrobronchoscope are hardly used outside the surgical area. VLs have been proposed as an initial approach by some authors, but their implementation is being limited and reserved as a rescue technique. It is true that these devices improve the vision of the glottis, but in less-experienced hands, they slow the procedure and, in critical patients with few reserves, additional few seconds can have fatal consequences.

## 6. Videolaryngoscopes in the ICU

In conventional airway management, routine OTI with traditional direct laryngoscopy (DL) is still the common practice [25, 26], with the Macintosh as standard gold DL, a device created just 10 years before the first ICU was Inaugurated by the anesthesiologist Bjorn Ibsen in Copenhagen (December 1953) [27, 28]. On the other hand, in DA cases, the technique of choice for intubation is the use of the fiber optic bronchoscopy (FOB), although there are more and more studies in which videolaryngoscopy is used as an alternative approach in induced/sleep or awake patient, since FOB is an expensive, fragile, and requires regular maintenance, is complex to dispose of in emergency situations or in prehospital emergencies, and requires previous training.

Failure of endotracheal intubation using Classical Direct Laryngoscopy with a Macintosh laryngoscope or other technique may occur unexpectedly. And, since the second most common event reflected in the NAP4 reports on the ICU was failed intubation, proper and correct use of videolaryngoscopes (VL) would offer the potential to reduce the difficulty of intubation in general in the ICU [1, 29].

Numerous studies have shown increased morbidity when performing multiple attempts at tracheal intubation. Videolaryngoscopes allow a view of the entrance of glottis independent of the line of sight (LI), especially those that have angled blades. The fact that the image sensor is in the distal part of the blade causes us to have a panoramic view of the glottis, without the need to "*align the axes*", thus avoiding hyperextension of the head, and in practice having a Laryngoscopy Cormack-Lehane (CL) grade 1 or 2 (CL 1/4 or 2/4) in 99% of the cases (**Figure 2**).

VL have also been shown to improve glottis and intubation success rates in emergency and emergency services, in the prehospital setting, and specifically in patients with known predictors of DA [30].

However, achieving CL grade 1 laryngoscopy (CL 1/4) in laryngoscopy with a VL does not guarantee the success of OTI, which is relatively frequent in VLs that have a curved leaf, especially during the learning stage [31, 32].

Previous studies with novice and experienced anesthetists have suggested that the learning curve with an optical device can be around 20 applications to be competent to manage [33].

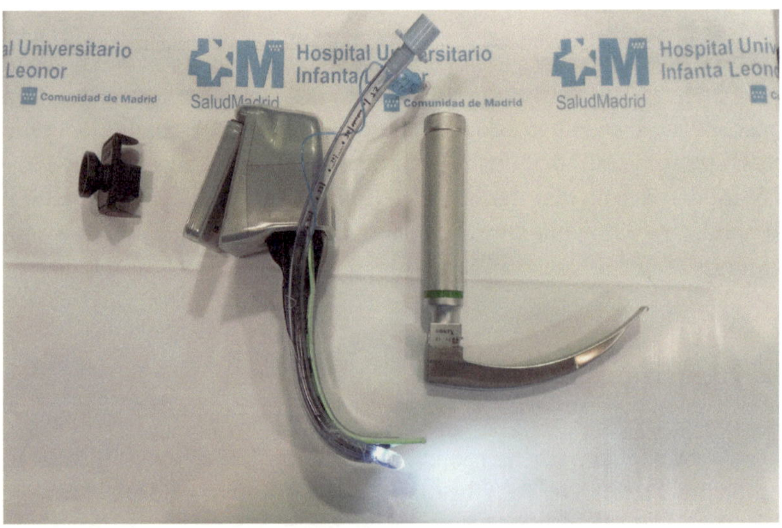


**Figure 2.** Glottic view differences.

Although these numbers are lower than those suggested by Greaves (80% of competence acquired with 30 cases, and complete with 100 cases), the video imaging technology of these new devices offers a shared vision between instructor and student [34], which can facilitate the teaching of airway anatomy, critical assessment of technique, and feedback. This may lead to skill acquisition faster than that achieved with traditional training with direct laryngoscopy [35].

This difficulty in achieving intubation despite the correct exposure of the larynx even in expert hands may be finally impossible, and success depends more on the operator's ability and patient's airway characteristics than on the own device [36]. However, in an attempt to overcome this problem, channeled videolaryngoscopes have the advantage of orienting the endotracheal tube (ETT) toward the trachea, allowing directed intubation with a little manipulation of the airway.

On the other hand, the evidence suggests that the use of indirect laryngoscopy (IL) improves the overall success rate of emergency/emergency tracheal intubation, as well as reduces the incidence of esophageal intubation when compared to conventional direct laryngoscopy (LD) [36].

In addition to this, we must mention that the VL, thanks to its good image quality, allow to easily recognize the structures of the larynx to achieve an image with a field between 45° and 60°, as opposed to the distant and tubular vision of the classical laryngoscopy (about 15°).

This image also allows to be certain about both the success of the intubation and the depth of insertion of the ETT, and can also easily recognize and correct esophageal intubation, a serious cause of morbidity and mortality. And another added advantage is that they provide an LED light, of greater luminous intensity than the conventional one and with a spectral irradiation closer to the human eye.

The NAP4 (the 4th National Audit Project on Major Complications in Airway Management in the UK) specifically mentions the theoretical benefit of videolaryngoscopes [1], with evidence that they can be more efficient than a Macintosh laryngoscope conventional.

For these and other reasons, these optical devices were incorporated into the airway management guidelines by the ASA as valid options in both the DA as usual, including, without excluding or limiting, laryngoscopes with different sizes and types of blades, VL, facial masks or supraglottic airway devices (SAD) such as laryngeal mask (LMA) or Fastrach® (ILMA), laryngeal tube, etc., fibrobronchoscope (FBO), extraglottic device (Frova, Eischman, etc.), nasal intubation, etc. [2].

### 6.1. Features

The characteristics that would define an ideal intubation device are described in **Table 1**.

During the last few years, many types of rigid, semi-rigid, optical, fiber optic and video-assisted laryngoscopes have been developed, as well as stiff and flexible stylets, as well as the classic flexible fibrobronchoscope, all of them with a common goal: to solve a classic problem for anesthesiologists, the difficult airway. The clinical evidences tell us about the real usefulness of all these devices in the solution of the problem for which they were designed. Scientific evidence of its use, the advantage of one over another, and the choice of each of them in a particular patient are yet to be determined.

| |
|---|
| • Light and portable. |
| • Economic and one-time use. Disposable, no risk of cross contamination. |
| • Short learning curve. Easy intubation with minimal skills. |
| • Good glottal visibility. |
| • Presence of an anti-fogging system that ensures the visualization of the airway despite the presence of secretions. |
| • Rapid orotracheal intubation, with minimal manipulation of the patient. |
| • Suitable for all types of ETT. |
| • Allow the administration of $O_2$/ventilate. |
| • Allow aspiration. |
| • It does not produce hemodynamic changes. |
| • Adaptable to the anatomy. |
| • Can be used with little mouth opening. |
| • Do not need cervical hyperextension. |
| • It can be used with the patient in any position. |
| • Possibility of connection to monitor for teaching. |
| • It can be used in awake patients. |
| • Multiple display options. |
| • Storage capacity and image integration. |

**Table 1.** Characteristics of an ideal intubation device.

At the moment, all the VL present as common characteristics [37–44]:

1. *Technically*: they present a wider image, high resolution, with improvement of the degree of laryngoscopy. Indirect vision of the glottis can be obtained in different ways:
   (a) Camcorder whose digital image is transmitted to a screen of an external monitor.
   (b) Beam of optical fibers.
   (c) System of prisms, which transmit the image through a system of lenses.
2. *Procedure*: similar to the Macintosh or Miller laryngoscope, although on other occasions it is inserted through the midline, or fiber optic bronchoscope (FOB).
3. *Teaching*: allow to teach and show multiple visions, the assistant visualizes and can see the result of laryngeal manipulation. The procedure can be saved and remembered. It facilitates the learning of alternative techniques to FBO, etc.
4. *Research*: images can be stored.
5. *Comfort for the user*: more comfortable posture, less contact with secretions, blood, etc.

### 6.2. Classification

Resulting the classifications proposed by Pott et al. [43], Healy et al. [38], and Niforopoulou et al. [44], although all VLs allow a view of the entrance of glottis independent of the line of sight (indirect laryngoscopy [LI]), could be classified according to the type of blade [42]:

1. VL with *"Standard"* rigid blade, similar to the LD Macintosh such as the C-MAC (Karl Storz, Tuttligen, Germany) or McGrath MAC (Aircraft Medical, Edinburgh, UK), among others. Also used as a conventional direct laryngoscope. This reduces, at least theoretically, the learning curve needed to use them correctly.

Other advantages common to all of them are the ease of visualization of the glottic structures, which allow to use any type of endotracheal tube (ETT) and the longer duration than the fiberscope, combined with the lowest cost.

The disadvantage is that, even in most of cases CL improves, the introduction of ETT is sometimes difficult and a certain practice is required, so eventually ETT must be performed with a guarantor (contrary to which occurs with angled blades).

2. VL with *Angled Rigid Blade* such as Glidescope (Verathon, Bothell, WA, USA), king vision with no channel blades (KingSystems, www.Kingsystems.com, distributed in Spain by Ambu a/S, www.ambu.es), the McGrath MAC X blade (aircraft medical, Edinburgh, UK), or the C-MAC D blade (Karl Storz, Tuttligen, Germany), among others.

All of them present advantages common to all of them: ease of visualization of glottic structures, allow to use any type of ETT and longer duration than the fiberscope.

The disadvantage is that, although Cormack-Lehane improves in most cases, the introduction of ETT is sometimes difficult.

The lack of a channel in which to put the ETT usually requires a certain practice and, often, it is necessary to preform the ETT with a catcher that provides the same the angulation that has the blade of the VL so as to be able to direct it to the entrance of the glottis.

3. Videolaryngoscopes with *Channel to guide* the ETT such as Airtraq (Prodol Meditec, Vizcaya, Spain, 2005. US Patent No 6,843,769), King Vision with a channeled blade (KingSystems), and the Pentax-AWS-S100 (Pentax Corporation, Tokyo, Japan), among others.

They all have a channel through which the ETT slides for intubation. As the ETT is directed by the channel, we must do any modification of movements on the device and not on the tube.

The tube does not need to be preformed with a stylet and generally enhances the Cormack-Lehane.

### 6.3. Current scientific evidence

The new optical devices are recommended to improve the management of the airway, both in anesthetic care and in critical patients [41, 42, 45, 46]. In recent years, the role of videolaryngoscopes has been debated, especially its use in the ICU [29, 31, 37, 42, 47–51], where there is a lack of scientific evidence and, in general, intubation is performed in more complicated conditions than in the operating room [52]. However, this evidence is supported in the surgical setting as there are randomized controlled trials (RCTs), meta-analyses, and systematic reviews. Although the environments are different, neither the techniques for the acquisition of competencies, and in one place as in the other, there are situations of unexpected vital commitment and/or deterioration of respiratory and hemodynamic function [7, 21, 41, 53, 54]. Therefore, the results of existing studies in surgical areas can be extrapolated to the field of ICU for many of the above-mentioned plots.

In this sense, Healy et al. published an updated systematic review of Videolaringoscopes in 2012 with the objective of organizing the literature about the effectiveness of modern VL in the OTI and then performing a quality assessment and making recommendations for its use [38].

The comparison of VL with LD was based on three main results: global success, first-attempt success, and successful intubation time.

The vision of the glottis was a desirable result, but since with the VL the intubation can be performed despite having a limited view of it and, on the other hand, a good view of the larynx does not always guarantee a successful intubation, it was not considered a target for the recommendation.

The final recommendations of the study could be summarized in three points:

1. In patients at risk of difficult laryngoscopy, the use of Airtraq, C-Trach, GlideScope, Pentax AWS, and V-MAC is recommended for successful intubation.

2. The use of the Airtraq, Bonfils, Bullard, C-Trach, GlideScope, and Pentax AWS by an operator with reasonable prior experience is recommended for successful intubation in CLD (CL $\geq$ 3).

3. There is additional evidence to support the use of Airtraq, Bonfils, C-Trach, GlideScope, McGrath, and Pentax AWS after intubation failed by direct laryngoscopy to achieve successful intubation.

Be that as it may, the use of VLs not only improves glottic vision, and in the ICU they also present other advantages such as positive effects on teamwork, communication and knowledge of the situation, as well as on technical skills. The use of VL on the training of residents, with an adjunct that shares their opinion as responsible for intubation seen on the screen, giving advice to help intubation, training nurses of the ICU allowing them to control the effect of the pressure on the cricoid during the sellick, adjusting it as necessary. In addition, the VL is immediately available, which means an improvement in the management of the unexpected DA [37, 55].

A major advantage of standard *"rigid"* VL, like the LD Macintosh, is that they use the same skills as LD, which reduces the need for specific training in VL, while facilitating the training of residents in the management of the airway by LD. In addition, intubation can be recorded for post-event teaching.

The study by De Jong et al., from the Montpellier group, evaluated the McGrath MAC (Aircraft Medical, Edinburgh, Scotland), a VL with a Macintosh type spade that allows intubation using conventional or indirect direct laryngoscopy. The results reported by these authors are similar to other studies, noting that it is easier to visualize the glottis using VL and that fewer attempts are required to achieve intubation. However, although De Jong et al. showed a significant reduction in the incidence of difficult laryngoscopy and/or difficult intubation with VL McGrath MAC (4 vs. 16%) in ICU patients did not provide information on whether or not actual intubation time was shorter [51].

In ICU, where patients are often under a cardiorespiratory compromise, reducing the time the patient is without adequate ventilation/oxygenation is probably more important than the time it takes to visualize the glottis. In the study by Yeatts et al. was found that a shorter time was required to insert an ETT when a conventional direct laryngoscopy was performed [56]. In fact, in this study, an IL with Glidescope (Verathon Médico, Bothell, WA) was associated with prolonged intubation times in trauma patients, with a longer time of hypoxemia and a higher mortality in patients with traumatic brain injury [57]. These results coincide with those of the ICU study carried out by Griesdale et al., who found that intubation with Glidescope VL resulted in lower oxygen saturations [58].

In addition, the study by De Jong et al., from the Montpellier group, evaluated McGrath MAC, a *"mixed"* VL that can be used both to obtain direct and indirect laryngoscopy vision [51]. This prospective study showed that systematic use of a *"mixed"* VL, also termed *"combo VL"* or *"combined VL"*, for intubation within a process of quality improvement using an algorithm of airway management significantly reduced the incidence of difficult laryngoscopy and/or difficult intubation.

In the multivariate analysis, the use of a standard laryngoscope was an independent risk factor for difficult laryngoscopy and/or difficult intubation, as was the Mallampati III or IV score and the status of nonexpert operator. On the other hand, in the subgroup of patients with difficult intubation predicted by the MACOCHA score (**Figure 3**), the incidence of difficult

| MACOCHA Score Calculation Worksheet | Points |
|---|---|
| ***- Factors related to patient*** | |
| **M**allampati Score III or IV | 5 |
| Obstructive Sleep **A**pnoea Syndrome | 2 |
| Reduced Mobility of **C**ervical Spine | 1 |
| Limited Mouth **O**pening <3cm | 1 |
| ***- Factors related to pathology*** | |
| **C**oma | 1 |
| Severe **H**ypoxaemia (<80%) | 1 |
| ***- Factor related to operator*** | |
| Non **A**naesthesiologist | 1 |
| **Total** | **12** |

Sources: De Jong et al. 2014a; 2013b

**M.** **Ma**llampati score III or IV
**A.** **A**pnoea Syndrome (obstructive)
**C.** **C**ervical spine limitation
**O.** **O**pening mouth <3cm
**C.** **C**oma
**H.** **H**ypoxia
**A.** **A**naesthesiologist Non trained

**Coded from 0 to 12**
**0 = easy**
**12 = very difficult**

**Figure 3.** Macocha score.

intubation was much higher in the standard laryngoscope group (47%) than in the "*mixed*" VL group (0%). These results were in agreement with the previous studies [51].

Cameron et al. perform a study to evaluate the odds of first-attempt success with video laryngoscopy compared with direct laryngoscopy, using a propensity-matched analysis to reduce the risk of bias, for intubations performed in a medical ICU. They accomplish an analysis of prospectively collected data for 809 consecutive intubations performed between 2012 and 2014 in the ICU of an academic tertiary referral center that supports fellowship training programs in pulmonary and critical care medicine [59].

This study comparing video laryngoscopy with direct laryngoscopy as performed by non-anesthesiologist trainees in a medical ICU demonstrates improved first-attempt success associated with video laryngoscopy. Author's findings are clinically significant and consistent with other reports and meta-analyses. These results, in combination with the existing literature on the success of video laryngoscopy and the availability of video laryngoscopy in most academic medical ICUs, suggest that video laryngoscopy should be considered the primary method of laryngeal visualization for intubations performed in ICUs, where there is increased risk of intubation-related complications.

A 2014 meta-analysis found that, compared with direct laryngoscopy, videolaryngoscopy improved glottis view and first-attempt success for orotracheal intubation in ICU [10]. However, both randomized controlled trials (RCTs) and observational studies were included in that study, and evidence from RCTs was limited. In the past months, new RCTs have debated the application of videolaryngoscopy in airway management in ICU [60, 61]. Bing-Cheng Zhao et al. performs a meta-analysis of RCTs to evaluate the effects of video laryngoscopy on first-attempt success and complications related to intubation in ICU patients [50].

Four RCTs enrolling 678 patients were included [60–63], and compared with direct laryngoscopy, videolaryngoscopy did not significantly improve first-attempt success rate (RR 1.17, 95% CI 0.89–1.53). In videolaryngoscopy groups, poor glottis visualization was less common (RR 0.30, 95% CI 0.14–0.64), and incidence of esophageal intubation was lower (RR 0.31, 95% CI 0.11–0.90). However, videolaryngoscopy did not reduce the time for successful intubation and other outcomes, including severe hypoxemia, hypotension, mechanical ventilation duration, and ICU mortality.

Nonetheless, trial sequential analysis showed that the current evidence on the use of videolaryngoscopy is still inconclusive. The prima facie question is whether there may be a type H error due to an inadequate sample size, seeing that there already exists a trend favoring the use of videolaryngoscopy in relation to the primary outcome of successful first-attempt intubation. A previously published meta-analysis of nine studies by De Jong et al. demonstrated the superiority of videolaryngoscopy versus direct laryngoscopy with an odds ratio (OR) of 2.07 (95% CI 1.35–3.16) [10]. Significant heterogeneity exists in the forest plot (P test 73%) with appreciable differences between the operators from inexperienced medical students to critical care medicine experts [50]. Nonanaesthesiologist as operator has been validated to be a risk factor for difficulty in intubation in ICU [64]. The operator's training and experience in comparative studies is, in our opinion, a critical factor which influences reported differences among various intubation devices. Out of the four randomized trials included for the meta-analysis [50], data from Silverberg et al. [61] was excluded for the analysis of time for successful intubation on the grounds of high bias risk (due to suboptimal allocation concealment and randomization strategy). The study by Silverberg demonstrated statistically and clinically significant differences in the time for successful intubation favoring videolaryngoscopy. Non-inclusion may affect the pooled data analysis by Zhao et al. [50]. Curiously, data from the same study was included for pooled analysis of the primary outcome (rate of successful intubation on the first-attempt). Two of the included studies compared the performance of the Glidescope with direct laryngoscopy, and two pooled data sets were included from studies comparing the McGrath videolaryngoscope against direct laryngoscope. Not all videolaryngoscopes are the same and the airway literature distinguishes channeled videolaryngoscopes versus the anteriorly angulated variety versus the Macintosh-like videolaryngoscopes—appreciating peculiar advantages and disadvantages of each. Combining results from all videolaryngoscopes as an entity may have its limitations.

In this regard, Joshi et al. [65] have tried to identify characteristics associated with first-attempt failure at intubation when using videolaryngoscopy in the ICU. They perform an observational study of 906 consecutive patients intubated in the ICU with a video laryngoscope between January 2012 and January 2016 in a single-center academic medical ICU. After each intubation, the operator completed a data collection form, which included information on difficult airway characteristics, device used, and outcome of each attempt.

In this single-center study, there were no significant differences in sex, age, reason for intubation, or device used between first-attempt failures and first-attempt successes. First-attempt successes more commonly reported no difficult airway characteristics were present (23.9%; 95% confidence interval [CI], 20.7–27.0% vs. 13.3%, 95% CI, 8.0–18.8%).

Presence of blood in the airway (OR, 2.63, 95% CI, 1.64–4.20), airway edema (OR, 2.85; 95% CI, 1.48–5.45), and obesity (OR, 1.59, 95% CI, 1.08–2.32) were significantly associated with higher odds of first-attempt failure, when intubation was performed with videolaryngoscopy in an ICU.

In a second logistic model to examine cases in which these additional difficult airway characteristics were collected (n = 773), the presence of blood (OR, 2.73, 95% CI, 1.60–4.64), cervical immobility (OR, 3.34, 95% CI, 1.28–8.72), and airway edema (OR, 3.10; 95% CI, 1.42–6.70) were associated with first-attempt failure [65].

There are important limitations in this study, such that when certain difficult airway characteristics such as blood, vomit, or airway edema could have been known before the intubation attempt or encountered during the attempt, it is possible that operator reporting of these difficult airway characteristics was more common when they were unexpectedly encountered. Moreover, multivariable analyses account for experience of the operator. The generalization of these study results may be limited given the exposure, airway curriculum, and experience of trainees at this institution compared to others.

Nevertheless, the intensive care professional should account for these difficult airway characteristics, blood, cervical immobility, and airway edema, when preparing for endotracheal intubation with video laryngoscopy in addition to standard practices employed to optimize first-attempt success.

Janz et al. [62] evaluates the effect of video laryngoscopy on the rate of endotracheal intubation on first laryngoscopy attempt in a randomized, parallel-group, pragmatic trial of video compared with direct laryngoscopy among 150 critically ill adults undergoing endotracheal intubation by Pulmonary and Critical Care Medicine fellows in a Medical ICU in a tertiary, academic medical center.

The primary outcome was the rate of intubation on first-attempt, adjusted for the operator's previous experience with the intubating device at the time of the procedure. Adjustment for the operator's previous device experience was performed by collecting the number of times the operator had previously used a VL or DL at the time of each intubation event during the trial, such that the adjustment for prior experience with a specific device was updated constantly as the trial progressed.

Videolaryngoscopy improves glottic visualization but does not appear to increase procedural success in unadjusted analyses or after adjustment for the operator's previous experience with the assigned device (OR for video laryngoscopy on intubation on first-attempt 2.02, 95% CI, 0.82–5.02, $p = 0.12$). Secondary outcomes of time to intubation, lowest arterial oxygen saturation, complications, and in-hospital mortality were not different between video and direct laryngoscopy [62].

The results of all of these studies are in contrast with results of prior studies demonstrating improved procedural success with VL [30, 36, 61]. There are several potential explanations for this difference, as that prior study limited to noncritically ill populations [66] may not apply to the patient, operator, and procedural conditions surrounding intubation in the ICU.

A lack of accounting of the experience of the operator at the time of the procedure [30, 36, 49, 61, 67] may also confound the results all of these works.

Several studies have shown that videolaryngoscopy enhances the laryngeal view in patients with apparently normal and anticipated difficult airways [32, 33, 39, 53, 68–70]. And there are a number of possible reasons why improving glottis view with VL does not translate into procedural success. Therefore, these data may not be generalizable to operators using videolaryngoscopes other than the McGrath MAC and direct laryngoscopes with straight blades. And some authors theorize that improving glottic view with VL may only matter to less-experienced operators [62].

The MACMAN trial (McGrath Mac Videolaryngoscope Versus Macintosh Laryngoscope for Orotracheal Intubation in the Critical Care Unit) is a multicentre, open-label, randomized controlled superiority trial published in JAMA [63]. It was a multicenter, randomized, open-label trial, which included all ICU patients that needed orotracheal intubation.

Lascarrou et al. try to determine whether video laryngoscopy increases the frequency of successful first-pass orotracheal intubation compared with direct laryngoscopy in ICU patients. They perform a randomized clinical trial of 371 adults requiring intubation while being treated at 7 ICUs in France between 2015 and 2016, and there was 28 days of follow-up.

The primary outcome was the proportion of patients with successful first-pass intubation. The secondary outcomes included time to successful intubation and mild to moderate and severe life-threatening complications.

The first intubation attempts were made by a nonexpert in 83.8% of patients. There were no difference in first-pass success between the VL (67.7%) and the ML (70.3%) groups (absolute difference, −2.5% [95% CI, −11.9% to 6.9%]; p = 0.60. These results were sustained even after adjusting for operator expertise and MACOCHA score.

The proportion of first-attempt intubations performed by nonexperts (primarily residents, n = 290) did not differ between the groups (84.4% with videolaryngoscopy vs. 83.2% with direct laryngoscopy; absolute difference 1.2% [95% CI, −6.3% to 8.6%]; p = 0.76). The median time to successful intubation was 3 min (range, 2–4 min) for both videolaryngoscopy and direct laryngoscopy (absolute difference, 0 [95% CI, 0 to 0]; p = 0.95). Videolaryngoscopy was not associated with life-threatening complications (24/180 [13.3%] vs. 17/179 [9.5%] for direct laryngoscopy; absolute difference, 3.8% [95% CI, −2.7% to 10.4%]; p = 0.25). In post hoc analysis, videolaryngoscopy was associated with severe life-threatening complications (17/179 [9.5%] vs. 5/179 [2.8%] for direct laryngoscopy; absolute difference, 6.7% [95% CI, 1.8% to 11.6%]; p = 0.01) but not with mild to moderate life-threatening complications (10/181 [5.4%] vs. 14/181 [7.7%]; absolute difference, −2.3% [95% CI, −7.4% to 2.8%]; p = 0.37).

The main reason for intubation failure in the ML group was inability to see the glottis, and in the VL group was failure of tracheal catheterization.

The ability to see the glottis is related to the expertise with the procedure and the equipment you are using, either way, since the groups were balanced regarding the physicians' expertise, the difference found between the two groups here might be because it is easier to visualize the glottis with the VL. The failure of tracheal catheterization, 70.7% (VL) vs. 23.5% (ML), can be explain with the learning curve or because they study a non-channeled VL. Eye-hand coordination, especially when looking through a monitor, is not learned with a few training sessions. Stratified by center and "*the status of expertise or nonexpertise of the individual performing intubation*". Unfortunately, the expert defying criteria did not include any experience with VL, and a good explanation for this difference is the lack of experience with the VL device besides the absence of channel in the blade.

Several studies comparing videolaryngoscopy with direct laryngoscopy have demonstrated improved rates of first-attempt success in the operating room, emergency department, trauma unit, and simulation laboratory, as well as during active cardiopulmonary resuscitation [56–58, 71–80]. Data comparing videolaryngoscopy with direct laryngoscopy on first-attempt success in the ICU are limited to a small number of observational studies [30, 36, 81–83], a meta-analysis of those studies [10], and some randomized controlled trials [60, 61].

Randomized controlled trial data comparing video laryngoscopy with direct laryngoscopy in the medical ICU are limited in number and external validity, especially for intubations performed by nonanesthesiologists.

### 6.4. Limitations

Videolaryngoscopes have among their disadvantages the cost, which mainly restriction access in areas outside the operating room. Devices need to be connected to the mains or batteries, and those that have an external monitor connected by cable may be little "*portable*".

Because they provide an indirect image, the blood, secretions, and fogging of the lens obscure the image.

The fogging can be prevented by pre-aspirating the pharynx, or by preheating or applying specific solutions to the distal lens if the device does not have a concrete anti-fogging system (such as GlideScope, Airtraq, King Vision, etc.).

Like any other device, VLs require a learning curve. Those who have a shovel similar to that of the Macintosh (without a canal) need a transglottic device (guarantor, Frova, Eschman, etc.), inserted through a technique that must be learned since they can generate traumatisms on the soft palate during its introduction. On the other hand, if the operator cannot properly position the device-channel blade, the tube can be guided into the esophagus. When this occurs, while maintaining a good vision of the glottis and the patient remains stable and well oxygenated, we can try to solve the problem by a light movement of the device (**Figure 4**) or the ETT (**Figure 5**), which will help guide the ETT and achieve successful intubation.

### 6.5. Complications

All of these devices allow an optimal visualization of the glottic anatomy, but sometimes the maneuvers required for intubation involve greater complexity because of the difficulty in orienting the ETT.

For this reason, specific guides and catheters have been designed for intubation.

Nevertheless, in parallel with the clinical use of these devices, complications have been described.

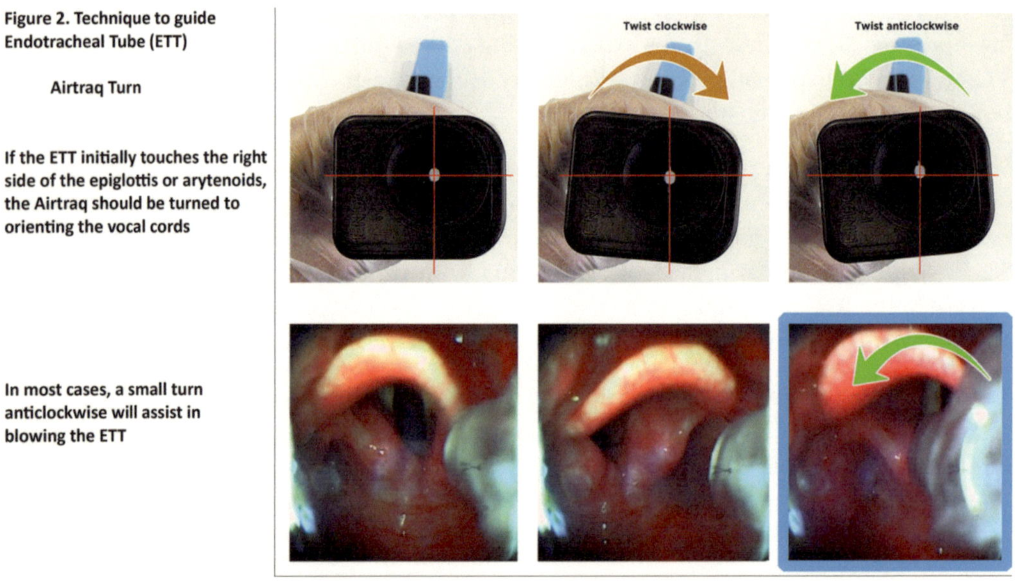


**Figure 4.** Technique to guide endotracheal tube (ETT).

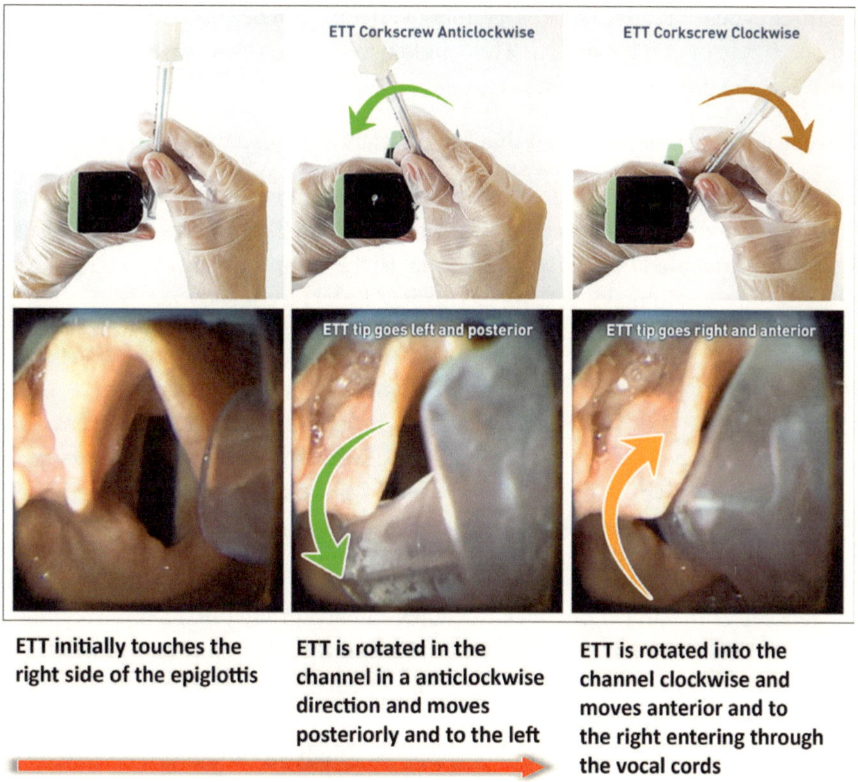


**Figure 5.** Technique for orienting the endotracheal tube (ETT).

Thus, lacerations of the glottic mucosa, vocal cord lesions, subluxations of arytenoids, and supracarinal tears are some of the complications encountered with the use of these new devices.

### 6.6. Practical approach to videolaryngoscopy

If we decide to use any device in our patients we think about practical approach of this device and not only in theoretical applications. In the case of videolaryngoscopes, we can raise doubts about how is the procedure different of direct videolaryngoscopy?

When we will perform the intubation, we must take into account that videolaryngoscope intubation is quite different than traditional direct laryngoscopy. The videolaryngoscope blade must be inserted into the middle of the mouth and rotated around the tongue in order to line up the camera lens with the larynx.

Always insert the videolaryngoscope midline into the mouth looking at the patient until its tip has passed the palate.

Once the blade has turned the corner into the pharynx, look at the monitor while glancing at your patient to optimally position the blade.

There are three types of blade. The non-channeled blades can be equal to the traditional direct laryngoscope blade or can be angled. This angle used to be 60° or similar, and make impossible direct visualization of the glottis.

The third type is the channeled blades that have a channel to lead the ETT toward to the glottis.

We have to be very clear that videolaryngoscopes allow a view of the entrance of glottis independent of the line of sight, especially those that have angled blades, but if we use a non-channeled and non-angled blade, it will be equal to the traditional direct laryngoscope blade, and we have a similar glottic view if we perform a direct laryngoscopy.

Other important question is about patient head position regard. One of the most important features of these devices, particularly angled blades, is that the head and neck should be in extreme sniffing position or in a neutral position during all the intubation intent. We can see indirectly glottis, independent of the line of sight, because the image sensor is in the distal part of the blade. This give us a panoramic view of the glottis, without the need to "align the axes", thus avoiding hyperextension of the head.

But, if we do not need to move head's patient, do we still lift the jaw upward like in direct videolaryngoscopy? In clinical practice, Cormack-Lehane grade obtained with videolaryngoscopes use to be one or two at last in 99% of the cases. But, this view not guarantees the success of intubation, which is relatively frequent in videolaryngoscopes that have a curved leaf, especially during the learning stage. This difficulty in achieving intubation despite the correct exposure of the larynx even in expert hands may be finally impossible.

So, in practice, sometimes perform the traditional maneuvers as lift the jaw upward, BURP maneuver, wear the epiglottis or move carefully the videolaryngoscope can facilitate the intubation.

As stated above, usually all patients had grade 1 or 2 Cormack-Lehane views (grade 1: full glottic view; grade 2: partial glottic view; grade 3: epiglottis visible but no glottic view; and grade 4: epiglottis not visible) with videolaryngopscopes. However, achieving CL grade 1 laryngoscopy in videolaryngoscopy does not guarantee the success of OTI, which is relatively frequent in VLs that have a curved leaf.

There have been a number of maneuvers suggested to increase the success of passing the endotracheal tube when glottic visualization is excellent and the tube is not easily passed using usual methods.

With non-channeled blades, once the blade is positioned with the larynx in view (as we explain in the previous point), we insert the ETT along the right side of the blade. Even though the magnificent view of the larynx on the monitor at this point, we must remember that the larynx is not in the direct line of sight.

Therefore, a properly curved stylet must be used to guide the endotracheal tube into the larynx. Unlike the typical "hockey-stick" shape used during direct laryngscopy and in the standard videolaryngoscope blades, the stylet should match the curve on the angled blades.

If it is being used a standard stylet, it must be placed into the ETT and then mold it against the blade so that the curves match. The ETT can leave into the sleeve to keep it clean.

http://dx.doi.org/10.5772/intechopen.72658

Because a standard disposable stylet is so malleable, occasionally it will straighten during insertion, especially if the oral space is tight. This leads to the scenario of being able to see the larynx and not being able to "get there". There are specific stylets, some of them nondisposable, which are preconfigured to the correct curve of their videolaryngoscope. Some of them are very stiff and can potentially damage pharyngeal structures, so that they must pull back slightly before fully inserting the ETT into the trachea.

Regardless of which stylet you are using, insert the endotracheal tube with the curve aimed toward the right side of the mouth, under direct vision until to see it on the monitor.

At this point rotate the tube back toward the midline, and aim it at the glottic opening.

If the mouth is small, it can be helpful to insert the ETT into the mouth first, slide it far to the right side of the mouth, and then insert the videolaryngoscope non-channeled blade midline.

To avoid lesions, it is mandatory to look at the patient during insertion of the ETT as described above until its tip has passed out of view beyond the tonsillar pillars. Only after the tip of the ETT has turned the corner into the pharynx should you look at the monitor, otherwise you can injure teeth, lips, tongue, and pharyngeal structures. Manipulate the tip of the tube through the glottis, and then pause to withdraw the stylet 2–3 cm. to effectively soften the tip of the ETT. Advance the ETT into the trachea looking at the monitor.

Channeled videolaryngoscopes have the advantage of orienting the ETT toward the trachea, allowing directed intubation with a little manipulation of the airway.

After successful intubation, remove the videolaryngoscope looking at the patient, not the monitor.

And, finally, we must think about regurgitation. Cricoid pressure, also named Sellick maneuver, is a standard anesthetic maneuver used to reduce the risk of aspiration of gastric contents during the induction of general anesthesia, applied after induction, in the period between loss of consciousness and placement of a cuffed tracheal tube. This is also a standard component of a rapid sequence induction technique. Cricoid pressure has been shown to prevent gastric distension during mask ventilation too.

A correct Sellick maneuver should be applied with a force of 10 N when the patient is awake, increasing to 30 N as consciousness is lost. These pressures occlude the esophagus and prevent aspiration during intubation, but often resulting in worsened glottis view and complicate intubation.

If initial attempts at videolaryngoscopy are difficult during rapid sequence induction, cricoid pressure should be released. This should be done under vision and suction available and, if we see regurgitation, cricoid pressure should be immediately reapplied.

## 7. Optimization of processes

In most cases, there is sufficient time to improve the intubation conditions, to perform an initial assessment and to evaluate the risk of intubation, to verify the availability of material, inductive agents and to plan alternatives.

Even so, on other occasions, the urgency of intubation in ICU is extreme (cardiorespiratory arrest, polytrauma, coma, etc.), and OTI should be performed in an optimal attempt of intubation with little time to optimize the patient.

Critical patient may present, mainly, hypoxemia, severe metabolic acidosis, hypotension, and right ventricular insufficiency [9, 16, 19, 20], with a degree of hemodynamic instability resulting in a low cardiopulmonary reserve, in addition to a full stomach, etc., and the implementation of a package of measures for intubation can reduce the incidence of life-threatening complications from 32 to 17% ($p = 0.01$) during intubation (biblioUCI46). This package of measures should consist of 10 key points (**Table 2**).

Of these recommendations, six have individually demonstrated their benefit, both in anesthetic practice and in critical care (noninvasive mechanical ventilation [NIM], the presence of two operators, rapid sequence intubation [drugs and Sellick maneuver], capnography, and protection ventilation pulmonary).

The presence of a second operator in crisis situations has been shown to reduce the complications associated with the OTI procedure such as esophageal intubation (0.9% vs. 3.4%), traumatic intubation (1.7% vs. 6.8%), bronchoaspiration (0.9% vs. 5.8%), tooth damage (0% vs. 1.0%), and selective intubation (2.6% vs. 7.2%). The overall rate of complications also decreased significantly (6.1% vs. 21.7%, $p < 0.0001$) [89].

**Prior to intubation**

1. Presence of two operators.

2. Perform a loading of fluids (500 ml of isotonic saline or 250 ml of colloid) in the absence of cardiopulmonary edema.

3. Preparation of maintenance sedation.

4. Preoxygenation for 3 min with noninvasive mechanical ventilation (NIMV) in case of acute respiratory failure (100% $FiO_2$, ventilatory support pressure between 5 and 15 cm $H_2O$, to obtain an expiratory volume between 6 and 8 ml $kg^{-1}$ and a PEEP of 5 cm $H_2O$).

**During intubation**

*Rapid sequence intubation* (RSI): etomidate 0.2–0.3 mg $kg^{-1}$ or ketamine 1.5–3 mg $kg^{-1}$, combined with succinylcholine 1–1.5 mg $kg^{-1}$ in the absence of allergy, hyperkalemia, severe acidosis, acute or chronic neuromuscular disease, burn patient of more than 48 h evolution and spinal cord trauma. Rocuronium bromide (rocuronium) 0.9–1.2 mg $kg^{-1}$ may be used when succinylcholine is not indicated [84–87].

5. *Sellick maneuver* [88].

**Post-intubation**

6. Immediate confirmation of the position of the ETT by *capnography*.

7. Noradrenaline if diastolic BP remains <35 mmHg.

8. Initiate long-term sedation.

9. Initiate *lung protection mechanical ventilation*: tidal volume 6–8 ml $kg^{-1}$. According to ideal weight, PEEP <5 cm $H_2O$, and respiratory frequency between 10 and 20 resp./min, $FiO_2$ 100% for a plateau pressure <30 cm $H_2O$.

**Table 2.** Package of measures for intubation in ICU.

Therefore, prior to anesthetic induction, at least the presence of two operators, water overload and preoxygenation with NIMV is recommended for 3 min in case of acute respiratory failure.

### 7.1. Patient's preparation

Before the AM should be prepared the basic material:

- Ventilation: facial mask of adequate size, manual resuscitator, oropharyngeal cannula.
- Intubation: laryngoscopes, videolaryngoscopes, endotracheal tubes, extraglottic devices (such as FROVA or an introducer of Eschmann).
- Position: the position of the patient is an important factor and limits the reduction of functional residual capacity. Several studies have shown that prior oxygenation in the semi-seated position or with the head at 25° can achieve greater $PaO_2$ [90, 91].
- Vacuum cleaner.
- Medication.

In the case of expected intubation difficulty, there should be a practically immediate availability of advanced AM material with different rescue devices of ventilation and intubation difficulty, as well as a Coniotomy cannula in the event of an eventual CICO situation.

The ICU should have prepared a difficult airway trolley, similar to those that can be found in the surgical blocks [1] (**Figure 6**).

### 7.2. Preoxygenation

Acute hypoxemic insufficiency is the main cause of intubation in the ICU.

One-third of patients had severe arterial desaturation ($SatO_2 < 80\%$) during intuation manevers.

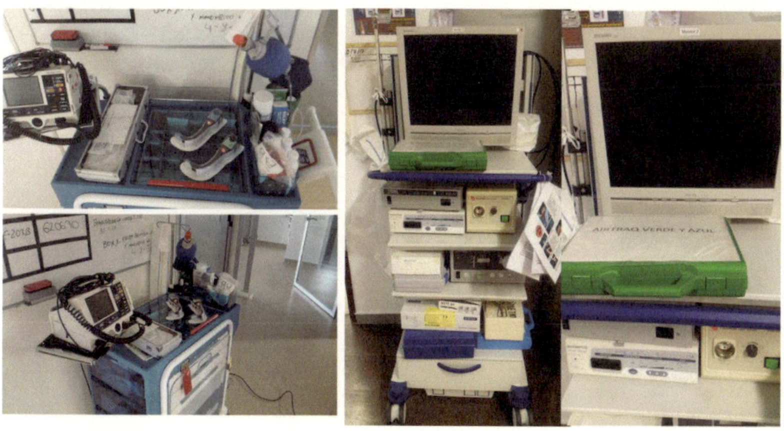

**Figure 6.** Reanimation difficult airway trolley examples. Left, Infanta Leonor University Hospital. Right, Getafe University Hospital, Madrid, Spain.

Hypoxemia may favor the complications observed during intubation such as arrhythmias, myocardial ischemia, cardiac arrest, and hypoxia in the brain.

Preoxygenation is the administration of 100% $FiO_2$ before induction. This maneuver aims to displace the alveolar nitrogen ($N_2$) by replacing it with oxygen (denitrogenation), in order to obtain an intrapulmonary $O_2$ reserve that allows the maximum apnea time with the lowest desaturation [92–96].

Traditional preoxygenation, performed with ventilation at current volume with Mapleson circuit and well-sealed facial mask, using a fresh gas flow of 5 L/min. of 100% oxygen for 3–5 min [94], is insufficient in the critical patient [97]. And only 50% of these patients will experience an increase of their $PaO_2$ higher than 5% compared to their baseline values after conventional preoxygenation for 4 min [98].

In all ICU patients, preoxygenation should be performed using a NIMV with PEEP 5–10 cm $H_2O$ + PS 5–15 with $FiO_2$ 100%, a management that has been shown to prevent patient desaturation during the procedure [98].

The mean pressure on AM will lead to alveolar recruitment, with the temporary reduction of intrapulmonary shunt [99] and an improvement in oxygenation. However, when this positive pressure is removed for OTI there is a risk of alveolar dis-reclusion, which will cause rapid desaturation.

Maintenance of continuous positive pressure during intubation with the use of a nasal mask has been shown to be beneficial in the operating room to patients with hypoxemic respiratory insufficiency and may be useful in ICU [100]. This apnea (or apneic) oxygenation is based on the alveolar pressure exerted by the blood circulation in the alveoli at slightly sub-atmospheric levels, generating a negative pressure gradient.

Another option is the high-flow nasal cannula (CNAF), a system that can provide up to 100% warm and humidified $FiO_2$ at a maximum flow of 60 L/min. [101].

This system allows an increase in $CO_2$ clearance due to better pharyngeal space clearance [102], in addition to the generation of a continuous positive pressure in flow-dependent AM (CPAP) (up to 7.4 cm $H_2O$ to 60 L/min), with the reduction of respiratory resistance and maintenance of alveolar opening.

### 7.3. Recruitment maneuver

Idea of NIMV use during preoxygenation is to recruit lung tissue available for gas exchange: "*open the lung*" with PS, and "*keep the lung open*" with PEEP.

The combination of preoxygenation/denitrogenation (with $FiO_2$ 100%) and the apneic period associated with the OTI procedure can dramatically decrease the pulmonary ventilation volume ratio, causing atelectasis.

Recruitment maneuver (RM) consists of a transient increase in inspiratory pressure, and there are several possible maneuvers such as applying a CPAP of 40 cm $H_2O$ during 30–40 s immediately after the OTI. When compared with not do, RM is associated with a higher $PaO_2$ (with $FiO_2$ 100%) 5 min (93 ± 36 vs. 236 ± 117 mmHg) and 30 min (39 ± 180 vs. 110 ± 79 mmHg) after intubation [103, 104].

### 7.4. Hypotension

Peri-OTI hypotension is a risk factor for adverse events, including cardiorespiratory arrest related to the management of AM, and up to 30% of critically ill patients may present post-OTI cardiovascular collapse [21, 54, 105–107].

Systolic blood pressure (SBP) <70 mmHg complicates 10% of intubations in ICU patients [9, 54, 106, 107], and when the patient has a preinduction gravity HR/SBP > 0.8, hemodynamic optimization should be performed pre-OTI and use inducing drugs with little response.

In responder patients, resuscitation with volume [108–110] can be made, while in the nonresponders, a perfusion of noradrenaline will be initiated [111, 112].

If pre-OTI resuscitation is not feasible due to the critical situation of the patient, vasoactive drugs will be prepared for bolus administration in order to maintain blood pressure during OTI and subsequent resuscitation. Although there is insufficient evidence, adrenaline diluted at a concentration of 1–10 mcg $mL^{-1}$, to be administered in boluses of 10–50 mcg, may be most indicated because of its inotropic effect [16, 109, 110, 113, 114].

In patients who are not in shock but exhibit a transient drop in post-OTI blood pressure due to the vasodilatory effects of induction agents or the onset of positive pressure ventilation, diluted phenylephrine at a concentration of 100 mcg $mL^{-1}$ will be administered in boluses at 50–200 mcg [16, 109, 110].

### 7.5. Severe metabolic acidosis

When acidemia develops from respiratory acidosis, it can be corrected rapidly by increasing alveolar ventilation. However, when acidemia depends on metabolic acidosis, maintenance of acid-base homeostasis depends on compensatory respiratory alkalosis based on alveolar hyperventilation.

In situations of severe metabolic acidosis such as diabetic ketoacidosis, poisoning salicylate, or severe lactic acidosis, the patient may not be able to make an alveolar hyperventilation that achieves buffering generated organic acids with a worsening acidosis [9, 16, 19, 20, 105, 115].

When OTI is required in these patients, even a brief apnea time can lead to a significant drop in pH given the loss of respiratory compensation that was already insufficient.

Therefore, OTI should be avoided in patients with severe metabolic acidosis in whom adequate ventilation with the ventilator cannot be ensured, and NIV can be used to adequately support respiratory work until correction of underlying metabolic acidosis.

If the OTI cannot be delayed, getting the patient to maintain spontaneous ventilation becomes a critical action during intubation and mechanical ventilation, as this will allow the patient to maintain their own minute ventilation. For this, agents with a low probability of generating apnea should be used. In addition, rapid sequence intubation should be avoided if possible, and if deemed necessary, a short-acting neuromuscular blocker such as succinylcholine should be used.

Once OTI is achieved, a ventilator mode should be chosen that allows the patient to establish and maintain their own minute ventilation to maintain respiratory compensation better.

### 7.6. Right ventricular failure

The main function of the right ventricle and pulmonary circulation is gas exchange. Under normal conditions, these are a low pressure and high-volume system which, in addition, must dampen the dynamic changes in volume and blood flow resulting from breathing, positional changes, and changes in left ventricular cardiac output. The adaptations needed to meet these conflicting requirements result in reduced compensation capacity in the event of a rise in afterload or pressure [105, 113, 116].

The failure of the system generates right heart failure, so that the right ventricle becomes unable to meet the demands, dilating, retrograde flow, decreased coronary perfusion and, ultimately, systemic hypotension and cardiovascular collapse [107, 110, 117].

When a patient with right heart failure requires OTI, increased afterload and decreased preload associated with invasive mechanical ventilation often leads to this cardiovascular collapse [21, 54, 105, 107, 113, 118].

In these patients, we should try to achieve pre-OTI hemodynamic optimization, including reduction of afterload with inhaled pulmonary artery vasodilators such as inhaled nitric oxide (INO) [119] or inhaled epoprostenol (Flolan) [113, 120].

In addition, good preoxygenation due to the reduction of intrapulmonary shunt [99], as well as apneic oxygenation [98, 106] will be essential, as well as avoid hypercapnia and high alveolar pressures, because they lead to vasoconstriction.

## 8. Critical airway management algorithm

As in the surgical setting, in order to limit the incidence of serious complications during OTI in the ICU, the entire process (pre-, peri-, and post-intubation) should be guided by protocols oriented to patient safety [2, 46, 121–124].

This critical AM algorithm will be based, firstly, on the outcome of the assessment of the difficulty of intubation according to the MACOCHA score [51] (**Figure 7**).

Always check the availability of the equipment for the AM and an eventual DA before the OTI. And, in the case of desaturation <80% during the procedure, the patient will be ventilated.

In the case of failure of intubation and ventilation, emergency ventilation through NIMV through a SAD allowing intubation [125] will be performed.

http://dx.doi.org/10.5772/intechopen.72658

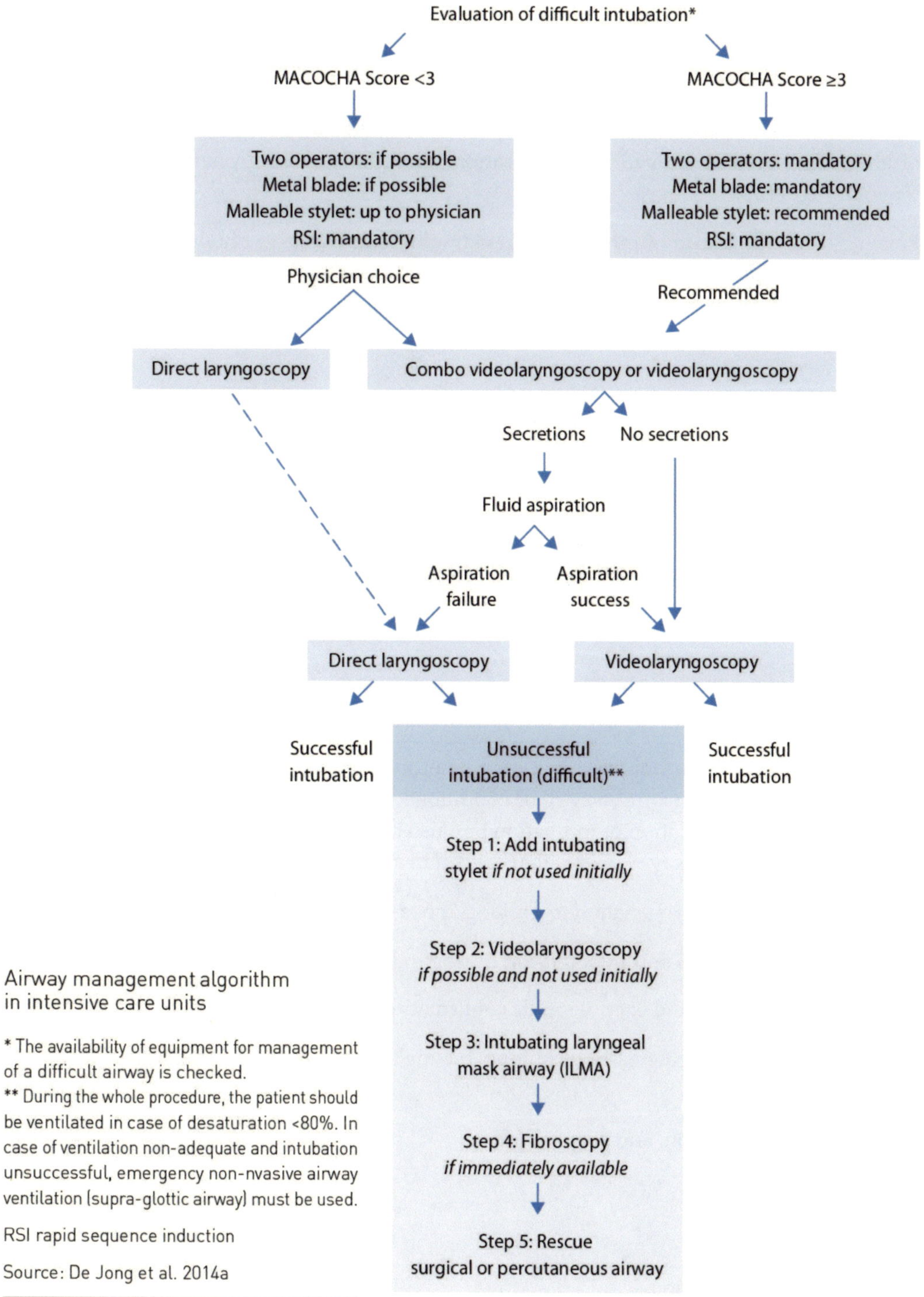


**Figure 7.** Macocha score protocol.

Two operators should always be present, especially if an AD with a MACOCHA score ≥3 is predicted, an extraglottic device (e.g. FROVA or an Eschmann introducer) should be used, and a rapid sequence induction be performed.

The use of a VL is also recommended in cases of difficult intubation. Nonetheless, in cases of abundant secretions, even after aspiration, direct laryngoscopy will be preferable to videolaryngoscopy.

Finally, in case of failure of intubation, an extraglottic device (e.g. FROVA or an Eschmann introducer) will be used first, followed by a VL if it was not initially used, rescue with a supraglottic airway device (SAD) that allows intubation, fiber optic bronchoscopy (FOB) and, at last, percutaneous or surgical rescue in situations of failure of intubation, ventilation, and oxygenation (CICO).

### 8.1. "*Not seemingly difficult*" airway management

It will be those patients who present a MACOCHA score <3.

The R rapid sequence induction (RSI) SI techniques are indicated in these cases, among others, in the ICU, hospital emergency services and out-of-hospital emergencies.

#### *8.1.1. Rapid sequence intubation*

The purpose of the RSI is to make emergency intubation easier and safer, and thus increase the success rate and reduce potential complications.

There is no single RSI technique due to its numerous indications, so the choice of the drug and the regimen of administration will be conditioned, not only by the reduction of the risk of aspiration and the facilitation of intubation but also by the characteristics of patient [88, 115, 126, 127]. However, the key elements that remain in all RSI protocol are:

- Preoxygenation/denitrogenation to prolong apnea time.
- Prevention of hypoxia and hypotension during induction and intubation.
- Use of a cuffed ETT, and capnographic confirmation of the placement of the tube.

In spite of the lack of a single RSI technique, the main steps could be summarized in [85, 88, 126, 127]:

- Valuation, planification, and preparation.
- Preoxygenation.
- Premedication.
- Induction and relaxation.
- Application of the Sellick maneuver.
- Laryngoscopy.

- Intubation. The RSI should allow us to intubate in a time no longer than 60 s from the administration of inducing drugs.
- Checking the placement of the ETT.

### 8.2. The anticipated difficult airway

Apnea following induction and neuromuscular relaxation may lead to rapid desaturation in the critical patient, if not in severe complications. In patients with previously DA [6, 40, 128, 129] or in those who were suspected according to a MACOCHA score ≥ 3, awake intubation would represent a valid option from the point of view of safety of the procedure [23, 29, 123, 130–133].

This intubation with the awake patient can be performed with a noninvasive technique or with an invasive technique (surgical or percutaneous), and among its advantages is that, by maintaining muscle tone, permeability of the airway and spontaneous ventilation, awake patients are easier to intubate because inducing general anesthesia tends to shift the larynx anterior.

The prerequisites for awake intubation in the ICU are:

- Previously difficult airway scenario or positive predictive signs (MACOCHA score ≥ 3).
- Patient cooperation.
- Equipment familiar with awake intubation techniques.
- Adequate AM preparation.

Contraindications:

- Human team inexperience.
- Negative of the patient.
- Allergy to local anesthetics.
- Hemorrhage in oropharyngeal cavity.

### 8.3. Difficult airway rescue

Before an intubation failure, we can find two possible scenarios:

- *Oxygenation with adequate face mask*: insisting repeatedly on a technique that has not resolved the situation will increase the risk of complications. Therefore, change to an alternative device (e.g. MCcoy blade), use an extraglottic device, use a VL, or a SAD intubation device.
- *Unsuitable oxygenation with face mask*: given the limited period of safe apnea of the critically ill patient, oxygenation, and not intubation, is the absolute priority in this scenario.

  There are different SAD that have been used to rescue ventilation with a difficult facial mask. The usual in ICU after ensuring oxygenation is that endotracheal intubation is necessary, so it is recommended to have some of the SAD that allow intubation through it [3].

  In the case of failure, a CICO scenario will be declared, the worst of the possible scenarios.

### 8.4. Can't-intubate-Can't-oxygenate scenario

CICO scenario is the end of the algorithms, and always constitutes a medical emergency that forces to explore an alternative plan based on transtracheal access, either through a percutaneous cricothyrotomy (choice for its speed), a surgical tracheotomy or through retrograde intubation.

This situation is reached when the attempt to AM had failed through tracheal intubation, facial mask ventilation, and a SAD. At this point, if the situation is not resolved quickly, hypoxic brain damage and death will occur.

The key points of the non-intubatable/non-oxygenable AM plan are:

- The CICO scenario must be declared and proceed to anterior neck access.
- A didactic technique has been described using a scalpel to promote standardized training.
- Placing an endotracheal balloon tube through the cricothyroid membrane facilitates normal minute ventilation with a standard ventilation system.
- High-pressure oxygenation through a fine cannula is associated with increased morbidity.
- All operators must be trained in performing a surgical approach.
- Training should be repeated at regular intervals to ensure that skills are not lost.

### 8.5. Adequate staff—adequate material—adequate procedure

Through the training program of those specialists who develop their professional activity in ICU must be guaranteed the acquisition of skills in critical patient's advanced airway management (**Figure 8**).

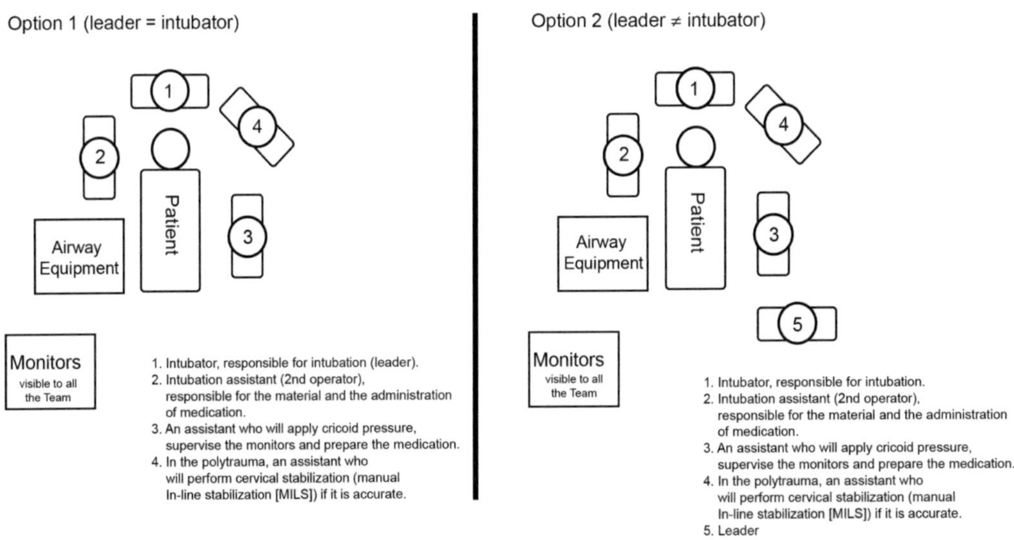


**Figure 8.** Teamwork, roles, goals and communication.

http://dx.doi.org/10.5772/intechopen.72658

Those responsible for the training of each service should develop training programs based on simulation to maintain competencies with different devices: direct laryngoscopy, extra-glottic devices, supraglottic devices, videolaryngoscopes, fiber optic bronchoscopes and cricothyrotomy set.

Also, each ICU should have immediate access 24 h a day to a difficult airway trolley that must include the same devices that the one usually available in the operating room.

## 9. Conclusions

Tracheal intubation in the critical patient is always potentially dangerous. Critically ill patients with acute respiratory, neurological, or cardiovascular failure requiring invasive mechanical ventilation are at high risk of difficult intubation and have organ dysfunctions associated with complications of intubation and anesthesia such as hypotension and hypoxemia. The complication rate increases with the number of intubation attempts. Videolaryngoscopy improves elective endotracheal intubation.

Every professional in ICU should have a basic knowledge about airway management, be familiar with algorithms to handle possible complications, and know correct use and interpretation of capnography. The algorithms that are usually handled by anesthesiologists in our routine clinical practice are not always useful in ICU because they contemplate alternatives such as awakening the patient or postponing the procedure that cannot be applied in a critical/emergency situation. The implementation of an intubation protocol in the ICU can contribute to significantly reduce the immediate severe complications associated with this procedure.

Airway management of patients admitted to the ICU is a challenge. New videolaryngoscopes have been proposed to improve management, but most studies comparing videolaryngoscopes with a standard direct laryngoscope (DL) have been performed in operating rooms. Therefore, the role of videolaryngoscopy in the ICU is still discussed, where there is a lack of scientific evidence and intubation conditions are worse than in the operating room. The Montpellier group has proposed and implemented a package for intubation care in its ICU which includes, among others, the use of two operators, fluid overload, preoxygenation, and, above all, the rapid detection of the position of the ETT by capnography. Including the use of videolaryngoscopy in this package, as described by De Jong et al. [51], the safety of tracheal intubation could be further improved.

The overall impact of VL on the anesthetic literature is weighed due to marked heterogeneity in the patient population, devices studied, operator experience, and confusion including manikin studies. While VL improves the ease of obtaining a view of the larynx, insertion of the ETT may be more difficult. VL may reduce the number of failed intubations, particularly among patients presenting with a difficult airway. They improve the glottic view and may reduce laryngeal/airway trauma. Currently, no evidence indicates that use of a VL reduces the number of intubation attempts or the incidence of hypoxia or respiratory complications, and no evidence indicates that use of a VL affects the time required for intubation [134].

The study of VL in the ICU is difficult for similar reasons, although they are increasing in popularity [10, 36]. However, there is a need for randomized controlled trials (RCTs) of VL vs. DL in the ICU [31], the truth is that the use of VL in ICU is so widespread that such studies are impractical. A RCT could help determine which devices are most useful, and could study the impact of VL on both technical and human factors [135].

If randomized controlled trials demonstrating a benefit of videolaryngoscopy are designed in the future, it could become a new standard for tracheal intubation in the ICU, particularly in educational institutions, where tracheal intubations are often performed by residents in training.

Nevertheless, the introduction of videolaryngoscopy in the ICU should always be accompanied by formal training programs in the management of the DA and simulation using manikins with the specific device [47, 71, 121, 136, 137].

Best way to avoid the serious consequences associated with a DA is the constant preparation by all those who could be able to handle it, an adequate prior assessment of the patient and the capacity to face this situation with the different rescue alternatives, from the use of SAD, VL, and flexibility in the use of the FOB, to the management of cervical surgical neck access.

Finally, we must implement the capnography in the ICU, so that the capnograph will be used in every intubation maneuver in the critical patient. Capnography should be monitored continuously in all critical intubated patients requiring assisted ventilation, and all ICU staff should be trained in the interpretation and recognition of abnormal capnography tracings.

In summary, if we consider the latest data, exclusive use of VL in out-of-OR airway management, or disdain them, appears premature, and we agree with the authors that future research would be necessary to demonstrate the safe utility of videolaryngoscopy in the ICU context. Even though it is surely the future to follow.

## Author details

Eugenio Martinez Hurtado[1*], Miriam Sanchez Merchante[2], Sonia Martin Ventura[3], Maria Luisa Mariscal Flores[3] and Javier Ripolles Melchor[1]

*Address all correspondence to: eugeniodaniel.martinez@salud.madrid.org

1 Department of Anaesthesia, Intensive Care Medicine and Pain Medicine, Hospital Universitario Infanta Leonor, Madrid, España

2 Department of Anaesthesia, Intensive Care Medicine and Pain Medicine, Hospital Universitario Fundación Alcorcón, Madrid, España

3 Department of Anaesthesia, Intensive Care Medicine and Pain Medicine, Hospital Universitario de Getafe, Madrid, España

## References

[1] Cook TM, Woodall N, Harper J, Benger J. Major complications of airway management in the UK: Results of the Fourth National Audit Project of the Royal College of Anaesthetists and the Difficult Airway Society. Part 2: Intensive care and emergency departments. British Journal of Anaesthesia. 2011 May;**106**(5):632-642

[2] Apfelbaum JL, Hagberg CA, Caplan RA, Blitt CD, Connis RT, Nickinovich DG, et al. Practice guidelines for management of the difficult airway. Anesthesiology [Internet]. 2003 [cited 2017 Aug 2];**98**(2):1269-1277. Available from: http://anesthesiology.pubs.asahq.org/Article.aspx?doi=10.1097/ALN.0b013e31827773b2

[3] Frerk C, Mitchell VS, McNarry AF, Mendonca C, Bhagrath R, Patel A, et al. Difficult Airway Society 2015 guidelines for management of unanticipated difficult intubation in adults. British Journal of Anaesthesia [Internet]. 2015 Dec 1 [cited 2017 Aug 7];**115**(6):827-848. Available from: https://academic.oup.com/bja/article-lookup/doi/10.1093/bja/aev371

[4] Rose DK, Cohen MM. The airway: Problems and predictions in 18,500 patients. Canadian Journal of Anesthesia [Internet]. 1994 May [cited 2017 Aug 7];**41**(5):372-383. Available from: http://link.springer.com/10.1007/BF03009858

[5] El-Ganzouri AR, McCarthy RJ, Tuman KJ, Tanck EN, Ivankovich AD. Preoperative airway assessment. Anesthesia & Analgesia [Internet]. 1996 Jun [cited 2017 Aug 7];**82**(6):1197-1204. Available from: http://www.ncbi.nlm.nih.gov/pubmed/8638791

[6] Krage R, Van Rijn C, Van Groeningen D, Loer SA, Schwarte LA, Schober P. Cormack-Lehane classification revisited. British Journal of Anaesthesia [Internet]. 2010 Dec 1 [cited 2017 Aug 2];**105**(2):220-227. Available from: http://www.ncbi.nlm.nih.gov/pubmed/21081683

[7] Frost PJ, Hingston CD, Wise MP. Reducing complications related to endotracheal intubation in critically ill patients. Intensive Care Medicine [Internet]. 2010 Feb [cited 2017 Aug 7];**36**(8):1438. Available from: http://www.ncbi.nlm.nih.gov/pubmed/7856895

[8] Le Tacon S, Wolter P, Rusterholtz T, Harlay M, Gayol S, Sauder P, et al. Complications des intubations trachéales difficiles dans un service de réanimation médicale. Annales Françaises d'Anesthésie et de Réanimation [Internet]. 2000 Dec [cited 2017 Aug 7];**19**(10):719-724. Available from: http://www.ncbi.nlm.nih.gov/pubmed/11200758

[9] Griesdale DEG, Bosma TL, Kurth T, Isac G, Chittock DR. Complications of endotracheal intubation in the critically ill. Intensive Care Medicine [Internet]. 2008 Oct 5 [cited 2017 Aug 2];**34**(10):1835-1842. Available from: http://www.ncbi.nlm.nih.gov/pubmed/18604519

[10] De Jong A, Molinari N, Conseil M, Coisel Y, Pouzeratte Y, Belafia F, et al. Video laryngoscopy versus direct laryngoscopy for orotracheal intubation in the intensive care unit: A systematic review and meta-analysis. Intensive Care Medicine [Internet]. 2014 [cited 2017 Aug 2];**40**(5):629-639. Available from: http://link.springer.com/10.1007/s00134-014-3236-5

[11] Law JA, Broemling N, Cooper RM, Drolet P, Duggan LV, Griesdale DE, et al. The difficult airway with recommendations for management—Part 1—Intubation encountered in an unconscious/induced patient. Canadian Journal of Anesthesia [Internet]. 2013 Nov 17 [cited 2017 Aug 7];**60**(11):1089-1118. Available from: http://www.ncbi.nlm.nih.gov/pubmed/24132407

[12] Law JA, Broemling N, Cooper RM, Drolet P, Duggan LV, Griesdale DE, et al. The difficult airway with recommendations for management—Part 2—The anticipated difficult airway Prise en charge des voies aériennes—2e partie—Recommandations lorsque des difficultés sont prévues. Canadian Journal of Anesthesia [Internet]. 2013 Nov 17 [cited 2017 Aug 7];**60**(11):1119-1138. Available from: http://link.springer.com/10.1007/s12630-013-0020-x

[13] Han R, Tremper KK, Kheterpal S, O'Reilly M. Grading scale for mask ventilation. Anesthesiology [Internet]. 2004 Jul [cited 2017 Aug 7];**101**(1):267. Available from: http://www.ncbi.nlm.nih.gov/pubmed/15220820

[14] Kheterpal S, Han R, Tremper KK, Shanks A, Tait AR, O'Reilly M, et al. Incidence and predictors of difficult and impossible mask ventilation. Anesthesiology [Internet]. 2006 Nov [cited 2017 Aug 7];**105**(5):885-891. Available from: http://www.ncbi.nlm.nih.gov/pubmed/17065880

[15] Kheterpal S, Martin L, Shanks AM, et al. Prediction and outcomes of impossible mask ventilation. Anesthesiology [Internet]. 2009 Apr [cited 2017 Aug 7];**110**(4):891-897. Available from: http://www.ncbi.nlm.nih.gov/pubmed/19293691

[16] Mosier JM, Joshi R, Hypes C, Pacheco G, Valenzuela T, Sakles JC. The physiologically difficult airway. Western Journal of Emergency Medicine [Internet]. 2015 Dec 17 [cited 2017 Aug 2];**16**(7):1109-1117. Available from: http://www.ncbi.nlm.nih.gov/pubmed/26759664%5Cnhttp://www.pubmedcentral.nih.gov/articlerender.fcgi?artid=PMC4703154

[17] Huitink JM, Bouwman RA. The myth of the difficult airway: Airway management revisited. Anaesthesia [Internet]. 2015 Mar [cited 2017 Aug 7];**70**(3):244-249. Available from: http://doi.wiley.com/10.1111/anae.12989

[18] Hung O, Murphy M. Context-sensitive airway management. Anesthesia & Analgesia [Internet]. 2010 Apr 1 [cited 2017 Aug 7];**110**(4):982-983. Available from: http://www.ncbi.nlm.nih.gov/pubmed/20357142

[19] Mosier JM, Law JA. Airway management in the critically ill. Intensive Care Medicine. 2014;**40**(5):727-729

[20] Griesdale DEG, Henderson WR, Green RS. Airway management in critically ill patients. Lung. 2011;**189**(3):181-192

[21] Mort TC. The incidence and risk factors for cardiac arrest during emergency tracheal intubation: A justification for incorporating the ASA Guidelines in the remote location. Journal of Clinical Anesthesia. 2004;**16**(7):508-516

[22] Sakles JC, Chiu S, Mosier J, Walker C, Stolz U. The importance of first pass success when performing orotracheal intubation in the emergency department. Academic Emergency Medicine. 2013;**20**(1):71-78

[23] Thomas AN, McGrath BA. Patient safety incidents associated with airway devices in critical care: A review of reports to the UK National Patient Safety Agency. Anaesthesia. 2009;**64**(4):358-365

[24] Miguel-Montanes R, Hajage D, Messika J, Bertrand F, Gaudry S, Rafat C, et al. Use of high-flow nasal cannula oxygen therapy to prevent desaturation during tracheal intubation of intensive care patients with mild-to-moderate hypoxemia. Critical Care Medicine [Internet]. 2014;**43**(c):1-10. Available from: http://www.ncbi.nlm.nih.gov/pubmed/25479117

[25] Kabrhel C, Thomsen TW, Setnik GS, Walls RM. Orotracheal intubation. Nejm [Internet]. 2007 [cited 2017 Aug 2];**356**(Anestesia, urgencias):1-3. Available from: http://www.nejm.org/doi/abs/10.1056/NEJMvcm063574

[26] Cooke H. Laryngoscopy: Time to change our view. Anaesthesia [Internet]. 2009 Apr [cited 2017 Aug 7];**64**(10):1143-1144. Available from: http://www.ncbi.nlm.nih.gov/pubmed/19317697

[27] Berthelsen PG, Cronqvist M. The first intensive care unit in the world: Copenhagen 1953. Acta Anaesthesiologica Scandinavica [Internet]. 2003 Nov [cited 2017 Aug 8];**47**(10):1190-1195. Available from: http://www.ncbi.nlm.nih.gov/pubmed/14616314

[28] Kelly FE, Fong K, Hirsch N, Nolan JP. Intensive care medicine is 60 years old: The history and future of the intensive care unit. Clinical Medicine (Northfield Il) [Internet]. 2014 Aug 1 [cited 2017 Aug 8];**14**(4):376-379. Available from: http://www.ncbi.nlm.nih.gov/pubmed/25099838

[29] Flavin K, Hornsby J, Fawcett J, Walker D. Structured airway intervention improves safety of endotracheal intubation in an intensive care unit. British Journal of Hospital Medicine (Lond) [Internet]. 2012 Jun [cited 2017 Aug 7];**73**(6):341-344. Available from: http://www.ncbi.nlm.nih.gov/pubmed/22875325

[30] Kory P, Guevarra K, Mathew JP, Hegde A, Mayo PH. The impact of video laryngoscopy use during urgent endotracheal intubation in the critically ill. Anesthesia & Analgesia [Internet]. 2013 Jul [cited 2017 Aug 7];**117**(1):144-149. Available from: http://www.ncbi.nlm.nih.gov/pubmed/23687228

[31] Larsson A, Dhonneur G. Videolaryngoscopy: Towards a new standard method for tracheal intubation in the ICU? Intensive Care Medicine [Internet]. 2013 Dec 12 [cited 2017 Aug 2];**39**(12):2220-2222. Available from: http://link.springer.com/10.1007/s00134-013-3118-2

[32] Bradbury CL, Hillermann C, Mendonca C, Danha R. Analysis of the learning curve with the C-MAC video laryngoscope: A manikin study. Journal of Anesthesia & Clinical Research [Internet]. 2011;**2**(10):167. Available from: https://www.omicsonline.org/peer-reviewed/analysis-of-the-learning-curve-with-the-cmac-video-laryngoscope-a-manikin-study-2124.html

[33] Falcetta S, Pecora L, Orsetti G, Gentili P, Rossi A, Gabbanelli V, et al. The bonfils fiberscope: A clinical evaluation of its learning curve and efficacy in difficult airway management. Minerva Anestesiologica [Internet]. 2012 Feb [cited 2017 Aug 7];**78**(2):176-184. Available from: http://www.ncbi.nlm.nih.gov/pubmed/22095109

[34] Greaves JD. Training time and consultant practice. British Journal of Anaesthesia. 2005;**95**(5):581-583

[35] Nouruzi-Sedeh P, Schumann M, Groeben H. Laryngoscopy via Macintosh blade versus GlideScope: Success rate and time for endotracheal intubation in untrained medical personnel. Anesthesiology [Internet]. 2009 Jan [cited 2017 Aug 7];**110**(1):32-37. Available from: http://anesthesiology.pubs.asahq.org/Article.aspx?doi=10.1097/ALN.0b013e318190b6a7

[36] Mosier JM, Whitmore SP, Bloom JW, Snyder LS, Graham LA, Carr GE, et al. Video laryngoscopy improves intubation success and reduces esophageal intubations compared to direct laryngoscopy in the medical intensive care unit. Critical Care [Internet]. 2013 Dec 3 [cited 2017 Aug 7];**17**(5):R237. Available from: http://ccforum.com/content/17/5/R237

[37] Karalapillai D, Darvall J, Mandeville J, Ellard L, Graham J, Weinberg L. A review of video laryngoscopes relevant to the intensive care unit. Indian Journal of Critical Care Medicine [Internet]. 2014 Jul [cited 2017 Aug 7];**18**(1):442-452. Available from: http://www.ncbi.nlm.nih.gov/pubmed/25097357

[38] Healy DW, Maties O, Hovord D, Kheterpal S. A systematic review of the role of videolaryngoscopy in successful orotracheal intubation. BMC Anesthesiology [Internet]. 2012 Dec 14 [cited 2017 Aug 7];**12**(1):32. Available from: http://bmcanesthesiol.biomedcentral.com/articles/10.1186/1471-2253-12-32%5Cnhttp://www.pubmedcentral.nih.gov/articlerender.fcgi?artid=3562270&tool=pmcentrez&rendertype=abstract

[39] Kaplan MB, Ward DS, Berci G. A new video laryngoscope-an aid to intubation and teaching. Journal of Clinical Anesthesia. 2002;**14**(8):620-626

[40] Hurtado EM, Pablo EL, Merchante MS, Flores MLM, Melchor JR, Cabezon NDL. Videolaryngoscopy Data Record. A Reality That Is Possible. 2015. Unpublished

[41] Hurtado EM, Merchante MS. Commentary to "Hemodynamic response to endotracheal intubation using C-Trach assembly and direct laryngoscopy". Saudi Journal of Anaesthesia. 2016 Oct-Dec;**10**(4):485-486.

[42] Eugenio Martínez Hurtado. Videolaringoscopios: Manual de actualizacion en Dispositivos Opticos [Internet]. 1st ed. Createspace Independent Publishing Platform, editor. Createspace Independent Publishing Platform; Edición: 1. ES; 2015. Available from: https://www.amazon.es/Videolaringoscopios-Manual-actualizacion-Dispositivos-Opticos/dp/1508874344/ref=sr_1_7?ie=UTF8&qid=1492155738&sr=8-7&keywords=eugenio+martinez+hurtado

[43] Pott LM, Murray WB. Review of video laryngoscopy and rigid fiberoptic laryngoscopy. Current Opinion in Anaesthesiology [Internet]. 2008 Dec [cited 2017 Aug 7];**21**(6):750-758. Available from: http://www.ncbi.nlm.nih.gov/pubmed/18997526

[44] Niforopoulou P, Pantazopoulos I, Demestiha T, Koudouna E, Xanthos T. Video-laryngoscopes in the adult airway management: A topical review of the literature. Acta Anaesthesiologica Scandinavica [Internet]. 2010 Oct [cited 2017 Aug 7];**54**(9):1050-1061. Available from: http://doi.wiley.com/10.1111/j.1399-6576.2010.02285.x

[45] Asai T. Videolaryngoscopes. Anesthesiology [Internet]. 2012 Mar [cited 2017 Aug 7];**116**(3): 515-517. Available from: http://anesthesiology.pubs.asahq.org/Article.aspx?doi=10.1097/ALN.0b013e318246e866

[46] Hurtado EM, Merchante MS, Flóres MLM, Saldaña PM, Escoda NA, Vecino JMC. Implantación de la Videolaringoscopia en la Historia Clínica Digital. 2015. Unpublished

[47] Manejo de la Via Aerea Evidencia Actual [Internet]. CreateSpace Independent Publishing Platform; Edición: 1. ES; 2017. Available from: https://www.amazon.es/Manejo-Via-Aerea-Evidencia-Actual/dp/1519140010/ref=sr_1_1?ie=UTF8&qid=1492155738&sr=8-1&keywords=eugenio+martinez+hurtado

[48] Hurtado EM, Merchante S, Melchor JR, Escoda NA, Cabezon NL, Saldaña PM. How Do We Face The Difficult Airway In Our Daily Practice? An International Survey. 2015. Unpublished

[49] Van Zundert A, Pieters B, Doerges V, Gatt S. Videolaryngoscopy allows a better view of the pharynx and larynx than classic laryngoscopy. British Journal of Anaesthesia [Internet]. 2012 Dec 1 [cited 2017 Aug 8];**109**(6):1014-1015. Available from: http://www.ncbi.nlm.nih.gov/pubmed/23154957

[50] Zhao BC, Huang TY, Liu KX. Video laryngoscopy for ICU intubation: A meta-analysis of randomised trials. Intensive Care Medicine [Internet]. 2017 Jun 4 [cited 2017 Aug 7];**43**(6):947-948. Available from: http://www.ncbi.nlm.nih.gov/pubmed/28260161

[51] De Jong A, Clavieras N, Conseil M, Coisel Y, Moury PH, Pouzeratte Y, et al. Implementation of a combo videolaryngoscope for intubation in critically ill patients: A before-after comparative study. Intensive Care Medicine [Internet]. 2013 [cited 2017 Aug 2];**39**(12):2144-2152. Available from: http://link.springer.com/10.1007/s00134-013-3099-1

[52] Cook T, Behringer EC, Benger J. Airway management outside the operating room: Hazardous and incompletely studied. Current Opinion in Anaesthesiology [Internet]. 2012 Aug [cited 2017 Aug 7];**25**(4):461-469. Available from: http://dx.doi.org/10.1097/ACO.0b013e32835528b1%5Cnhttp://search.ebscohost.com/login.aspx?direct=true&AuthType=ip,url,cookie,uid&db=mdc&AN=22673785&site=ehost-live

[53] Butchart AG, Young P. The learning curve for videolaryngoscopy. Anaesthesia [Internet]. 2010 Nov [cited 2017 Aug 7];**65**(11):1145-1146. Available from: http://www.ncbi.nlm.nih.gov/pubmed/20946399

[54] Perbet S, De Jong A, Delmas J, Futier E, Pereira B, Jaber S, et al. Incidence of and risk factors for severe cardiovascular collapse after endotracheal intubation in the ICU: A multicenter observational study. Critical Care [Internet]. 2015 Dec 18 [cited 2017 Aug 7];**19**(1):257. Available from: http://www.pubmedcentral.nih.gov/articlerender.fcgi?artid=4495680&tool=pmcentrez&rendertype=abstract

[55] De Jong A, Jung B, Jaber S. Intubation in the ICU: We could improve our practice. Critical Care [Internet]. 2014 Mar 18 [cited 2017 Aug 7];**18**(2):209. Available from: http://ccforum.com/content/18/2/209%5Cnpapers3://publication/doi/10.1186/cc13776

[56] Yeatts DJ, Dutton RP, Hu PF, Chang Y-WW, Brown CH, Chen H, et al. Effect of video laryngoscopy on trauma patient survival: A randomized controlled trial. Journal of Trauma and Acute Care Surgery [Internet]. 2013 Aug [cited 2017 Aug 7];**75**(2):212-219. Available from: http://www.ncbi.nlm.nih.gov/pubmed/23823612

[57] Taylor AM, Peck M, Launcelott S, Hung OR, Law JA, MacQuarrie K, et al. The McGrath® Series 5 videolaryngoscope vs the Macintosh laryngoscope: A randomised, controlled trial in patients with a simulated difficult airway. Anaesthesia [Internet]. 2013 Feb [cited 2017 Aug 8];**68**(2):142-147. Available from: http://www.ncbi.nlm.nih.gov/pubmed/23121470

[58] Malik MA, Subramaniam R, Maharaj CH, Harte BH, Laffey JG. Randomized controlled trial of the Pentax AWS®, Glidescope®, and Macintosh laryngoscopes in predicted difficult intubation. British Journal of Anaesthesia [Internet]. 2009 Nov 1 [cited 2017 Aug 8];**103**(5):761-768. Available from: http://www.ncbi.nlm.nih.gov/pubmed/19783539

[59] Hypes CD, Stolz U, Sakles JC, Joshi RR, Natt B, Malo J, et al. Video laryngoscopy improves odds of first-attempt success at intubation in the intensive care unit a propensity-matched analysis. Annals of the American Thoracic Society [Internet]. 2016 Mar [cited 2017 Aug 8];**13**(3):382-389. Available from: http://www.ncbi.nlm.nih.gov/pubmed/26653096

[60] Griesdale DEG, Chau A, Isac G, Ayas N, Foster D, Irwin C, et al. Video-laryngoscopy versus direct laryngoscopy in critically ill patients: A pilot randomized trial. Canadian Journal of Anesthesia [Internet]. 2012 Nov 30 [cited 2017 Aug 8];**59**(11):1032-1039. Available from: http://www.ncbi.nlm.nih.gov/pubmed/22932944

[61] Silverberg MJ, Li N, Acquah SO, Kory PD. Comparison of video laryngoscopy versus direct laryngoscopy during urgent endotracheal intubation: A randomized controlled trial. Critical Care Medicine [Internet]. 2014 Mar [cited 2017 Aug 8];**43**(3):717-718. Available from: http://www.ncbi.nlm.nih.gov/pubmed/25700064%5Cnhttp://www.ncbi.nlm.nih.gov/pubmed/25479112

[62] Janz DR, Semler MW, Lentz RJ, Matthews DT, Assad TR, Norman BC, et al. Randomized trial of video laryngoscopy for endotracheal intubation of critically ill adults. Critical Care Medicine [Internet]. 2016 Nov [cited 2017 Aug 8];**44**(11):1-8. Available from: http://www.ncbi.nlm.nih.gov/pubmed/27355526

[63] Lascarrou JB, Boisrame-Helms J, Bailly A, Le Thuaut A, Kamel T, Mercier E, et al. Video laryngoscopy vs direct laryngoscopy on successful first-pass orotracheal intubation among ICU patients a randomized clinical trial. JAMA [Internet]. 2017 Feb 7 [cited 2017 Aug 7];**317**(5):483-493. Available from: http://www.ncbi.nlm.nih.gov/pubmed/28118659

[64] De Jong A, Molinari N, Terzi N, Mongardon N, Arnal JM, Guitton C, et al. Early identification of patients at risk for difficult intubation in the intensive care unit: Development and validation of the MACOCHA score in a multicenter cohort study. American Journal

of Respiratory and Critical Care Medicine [Internet]. 2013 Apr 15 [cited 2017 Aug 7];**187**(8):832-839. Available from: http://www.ncbi.nlm.nih.gov/pubmed/23348979

[65] Joshi R, Hypes CD, Greenberg J, Snyder L, Malo J, Bloom JW, et al. Difficult airway characteristics associated with first-attempt failure at intubation using video laryngoscopy in the intensive care unit. Annals of the American Thoracic Society [Internet]. 2017 Mar [cited 2017 Aug 2];**14**(3):368-375. Available from: http://www.atsjournals.org/doi/10.1513/AnnalsATS.201606-472OC

[66] Su Y-C, Chen C-C, Lee Y-K, Lee J-Y, Lin KJ. Comparison of video laryngoscopes with direct laryngoscopy for tracheal intubation: A meta-analysis of randomised trials. European Journal of Anaesthesiology [Internet]. 2011 Nov [cited 2017 Aug 8];**28**(11):788-795. Available from: http://www.ncbi.nlm.nih.gov/pubmed/21897263

[67] Michailidou M, O'Keeffe T, Mosier JM, Friese RS, Joseph B, Rhee P, et al. A comparison of video laryngoscopy to direct laryngoscopy for the emergency intubation of trauma patients. World Journal of Surgery [Internet]. 2015 Mar 28 [cited 2017 Aug 8];**39**(3):782-788. Available from: http://www.ncbi.nlm.nih.gov/pubmed/25348885

[68] Sakles JC, Mosier J, Patanwala AE, Dicken J. Learning curves for direct laryngoscopy and GlideScope® video laryngoscopy in an emergency medicine residency. Western Journal of Emergency Medicine [Internet]. 2014 Nov 1 [cited 2017 Aug 7];**15**(7):930-937. Available from: http://www.ncbi.nlm.nih.gov/pubmed/25493156%5Cnhttp://www.pubmedcentral.nih.gov/articlerender.fcgi?artid=PMC4251257

[69] Maharaj CH, Costello JF, Higgins BD, Harte BH, Laffey JG. Learning and performance of tracheal intubation by novice personnel: A comparison of the Airtraq® and Mancintosh laryngoscope. Anaesthesia [Internet]. 2006 Jul [cited 2017 Aug 7];**61**(7):671-677. Available from: http://www.ncbi.nlm.nih.gov/pubmed/16792613

[70] Paolini JB, Donati F, Drolet P. Review article: Video-laryngoscopy: Another tool for difficult intubation or a new paradigm in airway management? Canadian Journal of Anesthesia. 2013;**60**(2):184-191

[71] Narang AT, Oldeg PF, Medzon R, Mahmood AR, Spector JA, Robinett DA. Comparison of intubation success of video laryngoscopy versus direct laryngoscopy in the difficult airway using high-fidelity simulation. Simulation in Healthcare [Internet]. 2009 [cited 2017 Aug 8];**4**(3):160-165. Available from: http://www.ncbi.nlm.nih.gov/pubmed/19680083

[72] Sakles JC, Mosier J, Chiu S, Cosentino M, Kalin L. A comparison of the C-MAC video laryngoscope to the macintosh direct laryngoscope for intubation in the emergency department. Annals of Emergency Medicine [Internet]. 2012 Dec [cited 2017 Aug 8];**60**(6):739-748. Available from: http://www.ncbi.nlm.nih.gov/pubmed/22560464

[73] McElwain J, Malik MA, Harte BH, Flynn NM, Laffey JG. Comparison of the C-MAC® videolaryngoscope with the Macintosh, Glidescope®, and Airtraq® laryngoscopes in easy and difficult laryngoscopy scenarios in manikins. Anaesthesia [Internet]. 2010 May 19 [cited 2017 Aug 8];**65**(5):483-489. Available from: http://www.ncbi.nlm.nih.gov/pubmed/20337620

[74] Kim HJ, Chung SP, Park IC, Cho J, Lee HS, Park YS. Comparison of the GlideScope video laryngoscope and Macintosh laryngoscope in simulated tracheal intubation scenarios. Emergency Medicine Journal [Internet]. 2008 May 1 [cited 2017 Aug 8];**25**(5):279-282. Available from: http://www.ncbi.nlm.nih.gov/pubmed/18434462

[75] Lim Y, Yeo SW. A comparison of the GlideScope with the Macintosh laryngoscope for tracheal intubation in patients with simulated difficult airway. Anaesthesia & Intensive Care [Internet]. 2005 Apr [cited 2017 Aug 8];**33**(2):243-247. Available from: http://www.ncbi.nlm.nih.gov/pubmed/15960409

[76] Savoldelli GL, Schiffer E, Abegg C, Baeriswyl V, Clergue F, Waeber JL. Comparison of the Glidescope®, the McGrath®, the Airtraq® and the macintosh laryngoscopes in simulated difficult airways. Anaesthesia [Internet]. 2008 Dec [cited 2017 Aug 8];**63**(12):1358-1364. Available from: http://www.ncbi.nlm.nih.gov/pubmed/19032306

[77] Mosier JM, Stolz U, Chiu S, Sakles JC. Difficult airway management in the emergency department: GlideScope videolaryngoscopy compared to direct laryngoscopy. Journal of Emergency Medicine [Internet]. 2012 Jun [cited 2017 Aug 8];**42**(6):629-634. Available from: http://www.ncbi.nlm.nih.gov/pubmed/21911279

[78] Aziz MF, Healy D, Kheterpal S, Fu RF, Dillman D, Brambrink AM. Routine clinical practice effectiveness of the glidescope in difficult airway management. Anesthesiology [Internet]. 2011 Jan [cited 2017 Aug 8];**114**(1):34-41. Available from: http://www.ncbi.nlm.nih.gov/pubmed/21150569

[79] Park SO, Kim JW, Na JH, Lee KH, Lee KR, Hong DY, et al. Video laryngoscopy improves the first-attempt success in endotracheal intubation during cardiopulmonary resuscitation among novice physicians. Resuscitation [Internet]. 2015 Apr [cited 2017 Aug 8];**89**(C):188-194. Available from: http://www.ncbi.nlm.nih.gov/pubmed/25541427

[80] Lee DH, Han M, An JY, Jung JY, Koh Y, Lim CM, et al. Video laryngoscopy versus direct laryngoscopy for tracheal intubation during in-hospital cardiopulmonary resuscitation. Resuscitation [Internet]. 2015 Apr [cited 2017 Aug 8];**89**(C):195-199. Available from: http://www.ncbi.nlm.nih.gov/pubmed/25541431

[81] Ural K, Subaiya C, Taylor C, Ramadhyani U, Scuderi-Porter H, Nossaman BD. Analysis of orotracheal intubation techniques in the intensive care unit. Critical Care and Resuscitation [Internet]. 2011 Jun [cited 2017 Aug 8];**13**(2):89-96. Available from: http://www.ncbi.nlm.nih.gov/pubmed/21627576

[82] Noppens RR, Geimer S, Eisel N, David M, Piepho T. Endotracheal intubation using the C-MAC® video laryngoscope or the Macintosh laryngoscope: a prospective, comparative study in the ICU. Critical Care [Internet]. 2012 Jun 13 [cited 2017 Aug 8];**16**(3):R103. Available from: http://www.pubmedcentral.nih.gov/articlerender.fcgi?artid=3580658&tool=pmcentrez&rendertype=abstract

[83] Lakticova V, Koenig SJ, Narasimhan M, Mayo PH. Video laryngoscopy is associated with increased first pass success and decreased rate of esophageal intubations during

urgent endotracheal intubation in a medical intensive care unit when compared to direct laryngoscopy. Journal of Intensive Care Medicine [Internet]. 2015 Jan 13 [cited 2017 Aug 8];**30**(1):44-48. Available from: http://jic.sagepub.com/content/30/1/44.long

[84] Seupaul RA, Jones JH. Evidence-based emergency medicine. Does succinylcholine maximize intubating conditions better than rocuronium for rapid sequence intubation? Annals of Emergency Medicine [Internet]. 2011 Mar [cited 2017 Aug 8];**57**(3):301-302. Available from: http://linkinghub.elsevier.com/retrieve/pii/S0196064410012072

[85] Lysakowski C, Suppan L, Czarnetzki C, Tassonyi E, Tramèr MR. Impact of the intubation model on the efficacy of rocuronium during rapid sequence intubation: Systematic review of randomized trials. Acta Anaesthesiologica Scandinavica [Internet]. 2007 Aug [cited 2017 Aug 7];**51**(7):848-857. Available from: http://www.ncbi.nlm.nih.gov/pubmed/17635392

[86] Álvarez Gómez JA, Ariño Irujo JJ, Errando Oyonarte CL, Martínez Torrente F, Roigé i Solé J, Gilsanz Rodríguez F. Empleo clínico de bloqueantes neuromusculares y su reversión. Recomendaciones del grupo de expertos de la Sociedad Española de Anestesiología, Reanimación y Tratamiento del Dolor. Revista Española de Anestesiología y Reanimación [Internet]. 2009 Jan [cited 2017 Aug 8];**56**(10):616-627. Available from: http://linkinghub.elsevier.com/retrieve/pii/S0034935609704785

[87] Tran DTT, Newton EK, Mount VAH, Lee JS, Wells GA, Perry JJ. Rocuronium versus succinylcholine for rapid sequence induction intubation. In: The Cochrane Collaboration, editor. The Cochrane Database of Systematic Reviews [Internet]. Chichester, UK: John Wiley & Sons, Ltd; 2015 [cited 2017 Aug 6]. p. CD002788. Available from: http://doi.wiley.com/10.1002/14651858.CD002788.pub3

[88] Algie CM, Mahar RK, Tan HB, Wilson G, Mahar PD, Wasiak J. Effectiveness and risks of cricoid pressure during rapid sequence induction for endotracheal intubation. In: Wasiak J, editor. The Cochrane Database of Systematic Reviews [Internet]. Chichester, UK: John Wiley & Sons, Ltd; 2015 [cited 2017 Aug 7]. p. CD011656. Available from: http://www.ncbi.nlm.nih.gov/pubmed/26578526

[89] Schmidt UH, Kumwilaisak K, Bittner E, George E, Hess D. Effects of supervision by attending anesthesiologists on complications of emergency tracheal intubation. Anesthesiology [Internet]. 2008 Dec [cited 2017 Aug 7];**109**(6):973-977. Available from: papers3://publication/doi/10.1097/ALN.0b013e31818ddb90

[90] Dixon BJ, Dixon JB, Carden JR, Burn AJ, Schachter LM, Playfair JM, et al. Preoxygenation is more effective in the 25 degrees head-up position than in the supine position in severely obese patients: A randomized controlled study. Anesthesiology [Internet]. 2005 Jun [cited 2017 Aug 7];**102**(6):1110-1115; discussion 5A. Available from: http://www.ncbi.nlm.nih.gov/pubmed/15915022

[91] Ramkumar V, Umesh G, Ann Philip F. Preoxygenation with 20° head-up tilt provides longer duration of non-hypoxic apnea than conventional preoxygenation in non-obese healthy adults. Journal of Anesthesia [Internet]. 2011 Apr 4 [cited 2017 Aug 7];**25**(2):189-194. Available from: http://www.ncbi.nlm.nih.gov/pubmed/21293885

[92] Norris MC, Kirkland MR, Torjman MC, Goldberg ME. Denitrogenation in pregnancy. Canadian Journal of Anesthesia [Internet]. 1989 Sep [cited 2017 Aug 7];**36**(5):523-525. Available from: http://www.ncbi.nlm.nih.gov/pubmed/2791175

[93] Carmichael FJ, Cruise CJE. Preoxygenation—A study of denitrogenation.pdf. Obstetric Anesthesia Digest [Internet]. 1989 Mar [cited 2017 Aug 7];**68**(3):406-409. Available from: http://www.ncbi.nlm.nih.gov/pubmed/2493208

[94] Hubert S, Massa H, Ruggiu G, Raucoules-Aimé M. Preoxigenación en anestesia. EMC—Anestesia-Reanimación. 2009;**35**(3):1-6.

[95] Preoxygenation: Physiology and practice. Lancet [Internet]. 1992 Jan 4 [cited 2017 Aug 7]; **339**(8784):31-32. Available from: http://www.ncbi.nlm.nih.gov/pubmed/1345958

[96] De Jong A, Futier E, Millot A, Coisel Y, Jung B, Chanques G, et al. How to preoxygenate in operative room: healthy subjects and situations "at risk." Annales Françaises D'anesthèsie et de Rèanimation [Internet]. 2014 Jul [cited 2017 Aug 7];**33**(7-8):457-461. Available from: http://www.ncbi.nlm.nih.gov/pubmed/25168301

[97] Mort TC. Preoxygenation in critically ill patients requiring emergency tracheal intubation. Critical Care Medicine [Internet]. 2005 Nov [cited 2017 Aug 7];**33**(11):2672-2675. Available from: http://www.ncbi.nlm.nih.gov/entrez/query.fcgi?cmd=Retrieve&db=PubMed&dopt=Citation&list_uids=16276196

[98] Baillard C, Fosse JP, Sebbane M, Chanques G, Vincent F, Courouble P, et al. Noninvasive ventilation improves preoxygenation before intubation of hypoxic patients. American Journal of Respiratory and Critical Care Medicine [Internet]. 2006 Jul 15 [cited 2017 Aug 7];**174**(2):171-177. Available from: http://www.ncbi.nlm.nih.gov/pubmed/16627862

[99] Findley LJ, Ries AL, Tisi GM, Wagner PD. Hypoxemia during apnea in normal subjects: Mechanisms and impact of lung volume. Journal of Applied Physiology [Internet]. 1983 Dec [cited 2017 Aug 7];**55**(6):1777-1783. Available from: http://www.ncbi.nlm.nih.gov/pubmed/6662768

[100] Barjaktarevic I, Berlin D. Bronchoscopic intubation during continuous nasal positive pressure ventilation in the treatment of hypoxemic respiratory failure. Journal of Intensive Care Medicine [Internet]. 2013 Mar 15 [cited 2017 Aug 7];**30**(3):161-166. Available from: http://www.ncbi.nlm.nih.gov/pubmed/24243561

[101] Ricard J-D. High flow nasal oxygen in acute respiratory failure. Minerva Anestesiologica [Internet]. 2012 Jul [cited 2017 Aug 8];**78**(7):836-841. Available from: http://www.ncbi.nlm.nih.gov/pubmed/22531566

[102] Vourc'h M, Asfar P, Volteau C, Bachoumas K, Clavieras N, Egreteau PY, et al. High-flow nasal cannula oxygen during endotracheal intubation in hypoxemic patients: A randomized controlled clinical trial. Intensive Care Medicine [Internet]. 2015 Sep [cited 2017 Aug 7];**41**(9):1538-1548. Available from: http://www.ncbi.nlm.nih.gov/pubmed/25869405

[103] Constantin J-M, Futier E, Cherprenet A-L, Chanques G, Guerin R, Cayot-Constantin S, et al. A recruitment maneuver increases oxygenation after intubation of hypoxemic intensive

care unit patients: a randomized controlled study. Critical Care [Internet]. 2010 [cited 2017 Aug 7];**14**(2):R76. Available from: http://www.ncbi.nlm.nih.gov/pubmed/20426859

[104] Futier E, Constantin J-M, Petit A, Jung B, Kwiatkowski F, Duclos M, et al. Positive end-expiratory pressure improves end-expiratory lung volume but not oxygenation after induction of anaesthesia. European Journal of Anaesthesiology [Internet]. 2010 Apr [cited 2017 Aug 7];**27**(6):508-513. Available from: http://www.ncbi.nlm.nih.gov/pubmed/20404729

[105] Haddad F, Hunt SA, Rosenthal DN, Murphy DJ. Right ventricular function in cardiovascular disease, part I: Anatomy, physiology, aging, and functional assessment of the right ventricle. Circulation [Internet]. 2008 Mar 18 [cited 2017 Aug 7];**117**(11):1436-1448. Available from: http://www.ncbi.nlm.nih.gov/pubmed/18347220

[106] Dewhirst E, Frazier WJ, Leder M, Fraser DD, Tobias JD. Cardiac arrest following ketamine administration for rapid sequence intubation. Journal of Intensive Care Medicine [Internet]. 2012 Nov 29 [cited 2017 Aug 7];**28**(6):375-379. Available from: http://www.ncbi.nlm.nih.gov/pubmed/22644454

[107] Martinez Hurtado E, Sanchez Merchante M. Commentary to "Hemodynamic response to endotracheal intubation using C-Trach assembly and direct laryngoscopy". Saudi Journal of Anaesthesia [serial online] 2016 [cited 2017 Nov 22];**10**:485-486. Available from: http://europepmc.org/abstract/med/27833506

[108] De Backer D, Biston P, Devriendt J, Madl C, Chochrad D, Aldecoa C, et al. Comparison of dopamine and norepinephrine in the treatment of shock. New England Journal of Medicine [Internet]. 2010 Mar 4 [cited 2017 Aug 7];**362**(9):779-789. Available from: http://www.ncbi.nlm.nih.gov/pubmed/20200382

[109] Ripollés-Melchor J, Casans-Francés R, Espinosa A, Abad-Gurumeta A, Feldheiser A, López-Timoneda F, et al. Goal directed hemodynamic therapy based in esophageal Doppler flow parameters: A systematic review, meta-analysis and trial sequential analysis. Revista Española de Anestesiología y Reanimación (English Ed). 2016 Aug-Sep;**63**(7):384-405. doi: 10.1016/j.redar.2015.07.009. Epub 2016 Feb 10

[110] Ripollés J, Espinosa A, Martínez-Hurtado E, Abad-Gurumeta A, Casans-Francés R, Fernández-Pérez C, et al. Intraoperative goal directed hemodynamic therapy in noncardiac surgery: A systematic review and meta-analysis | Terapia hemodinâmica alvo-dirigida no intraoperatório de cirurgia não cardíaca: revisão sistemática e meta-análise. Brazilian Journal of Anesthesiology [Internet]. 2016 Sep-Oct;**66**(5):513-528. doi: 10.1016/j.bjane.2015.02.001. Epub 2015 Sep 14

[111] Monnet X, Letierce A, Hamzaoui O, Chemla D, Anguel N, Osman D, et al. Arterial pressure allows monitoring the changes in cardiac output induced by volume expansion but not by norepinephrine. Critical Care Med [Internet]. 2011 Jun [cited 2017 Aug 7];**39**(6):1394-1399. Available from: http://www.ncbi.nlm.nih.gov/pubmed/21336124

[112] Loubani OM, Green RS. A systematic review of extravasation and local tissue injury from administration of vasopressors through peripheral intravenous catheters and central

venous catheters. Journal of Critical Care [Internet]. 2015 Jun [cited 2017 Aug 7];**30**(3):653.e9-653.e17. Available from: http://www.ncbi.nlm.nih.gov/pubmed/25669592

[113] Krishnan S, Schmidt GA. Acute right ventricular dysfunction: Real-time management with echocardiography. Chest [Internet]. 2015 Mar [cited 2017 Aug 7];**147**(3):835-846. Available from: http://www.ncbi.nlm.nih.gov/pubmed/25732449

[114] Calvo-Vecino JM, Hernández EV, Rodríguez JMR, Segurola CL, Trapero CM, Quintas CN, et al. Vía Clínica de Recuperación Intensificada en Cirugía Abdominal (RICA). Instituto Aragonés de Ciencias de la Salud. 2014.

[115] Leeuwenburg T. Airway management of the critically ill patient: Modifications of traditional rapid sequence induction and intubation. Critical Care Horizons [Internet]. 2015;**1**(1):1-10. Available from: http://www.criticalcarehorizons.com/wp-content/uploads/2014/06/airway-management-critically.pdf

[116] Greyson CR. Ventrículo derecho y circulación pulmonar: Conceptos básicos. Revista Española de Cardiología [Internet]. 2010 [cited 2017 Aug 2];**63**(1):81-95. Available from: http://linkinghub.elsevier.com/retrieve/pii/S0300893210700129

[117] Lupi-Herrera E, Santos Martínez L-E, Figueroa Solano J, Sandoval Zárate J. [Homeometric autoregulation in the heart. The Anrep effect. Its possible role in increased right ventricular afterload pathophysiology]. Archivos de Cardiologia de Mexico [Internet]. [cited 2017 Aug 7];**77**(4):330-348. Available from: http://www.ncbi.nlm.nih.gov/pubmed/18361080

[118] Dalabih M, Rischard F, Mosier JM. What´s new: The management of acute right ventricular decompensation of chronic pulmonary hypertension. Intensive Care Medicine [Internet]. 2014 Dec 3 [cited 2017 Aug 7];**40**(12):1930-1933. Available from: http://www.ncbi.nlm.nih.gov/pubmed/25183571

[119] Germann P, Braschi A, Della Rocca G, Dinh-Xuan AT, Falke K, Frostell C, et al. Inhaled nitric oxide therapy in adults: European expert recommendations. Intensive Care Medicine [Internet]. 2005 Aug 23 [cited 2017 Aug 7];**31**(8):1029-1041. Available from: http://www.ncbi.nlm.nih.gov/pubmed/15973521

[120] Howell JB, Permutt S, Proctor DF, Riley RL. Effect of inflation of the lung on different parts of pulmonary vascular bed. Journal of Applied Physiology [Internet]. 1961 Jan [cited 2017 Aug 7];**16**:71-76. Available from: http://www.ncbi.nlm.nih.gov/pubmed/13716268

[121] Jaber S, Jung B, Corne P, Sebbane M, Muller L, Chanques G, et al. An intervention to decrease complications related to endotracheal intubation in the intensive care unit: A prospective, multiple-center study. Intensive Care Medicine [Internet]. 2010 Feb 17 [cited 2017 Aug 7];**36**(2):248-255. Available from: http://www.ncbi.nlm.nih.gov/pubmed/19921148

[122] Langeron O, Amour J, Vivien B, Aubrun F. Clinical review: Management of difficult airways. Critical Care. 2006;**10**(6):243

[123] Mariscal Flores M, Martínez Hurtado E, Cuesta R, Jiménez MJ. ¿Existe un Gold Standard en el manejo de la VAD? Revisión 2015. Revista Electrónica de AnestesiaR [Internet]. 2016;**8**(2):384. Available from: http://anestesiar.org/rear/volumen-viii-2016/numero-02/659-existe-un-gold-standard-en-el-manejo-de-la-via-aerea-dificil-revision-2015

[124] Serocki G, Bein B, Scholz J, Dörges V. Management of the predicted difficult airway: A comparison of conventional blade laryngoscopy with video-assisted blade laryngoscopy and the GlideScope. European Journal of Anaesthesiology. 2010;**27**(1):24-30.

[125] Mariscal Flores M, Martinez Hurtado E. Platform CIP, editor. Actualizaciones en VAD: Puesta al dia—2014-2015 [Internet]. 1st ed. AnestesiaR; 2014. 274 p. Available from: https://www.amazon.es/Actualizaciones-Via-Aerea-Dificil-Puesta/dp/1503008037

[126] Palencia-Herrejon E, Borrallo-Perez JM, Pardo-Rey C. Intubation of the critical patient. Medicina Intensiva. 2008;**32**(1):3-11

[127] Fenwick R. Rapid sequence induction in urgent care settings. Emergency Nurse [Internet]. 2014 Mar 5 [cited 2017 Aug 7];**21**(10):16-24. Available from: http://www.ncbi.nlm.nih.gov/pubmed/24597816

[128] Cormack RS, Lehane J. Difficult tracheal intubation in obstetrics. Anaesthesia. 1984;**39**(11):1105-1111

[129] Pearce A. Evaluation of the airway and preparation for difficulty. Best Practice & Research Clinical Anaesthesiology [Internet]. 2005 Dec [cited 2017 Aug 7];**19**(4):559-579. Available from: http://www.ncbi.nlm.nih.gov/pubmed/16408534

[130] Brichant JF. [The Helsinki declaration on patient safety in anaesthesiology]. Acta Anaesthesiologica Belgica [Internet]. 2010 Jul [cited 2017 Aug 7];**61**(2):49. Available from: http://content.wkhealth.com/linkback/openurl?sid=WKPTLP:landingpage&an=00003643-201007000-00003

[131] Valero R, Sabaté S, Borràs R, Áñez C, Bermejo S, González-Carrasco FJ, Andreu E, Villalonga R, López A, Villalonga A, Massó E. Secció de Via Aèria de la Societat Catalana d'Anestesiologia, Reanimació i Terapèutica del Dolor. Recomendaciones sobre seguridad del paciente quirúrgico. Protocolo de manejo de la vía aérea difícil. Implicación de la Declaración de Helsinki. Difficult airway management protocol. Involvement of the Declaration of Helsinki. Revista Española de Anestesiología y Reanimación [Internet]. 2013;**60**(Supl 1):34-45. DOI: 10.1016/S0034-9356(13)70008-2 (https://goo.gl/7zpeFn)

[132] Woodall N, Frerk C, Cook TM. Can we make airway management (even) safer?—Lessons from national audit. Anaesthesia [Internet]. 2011 Dec [cited 2017 Aug 7];**66**(Suppl. 2):27-33. Available from: http://www.ncbi.nlm.nih.gov/pubmed/22074076

[133] Metzner J, Posner KL, Lam MS, Domino KB. Closed claims' analysis. Best Practice & Research Clinical Anaesthesiology. 2011;**25**(2):263-276

[134] Lewis SR, Butler AR, Parker J, Cook TM, Smith AF. Videolaryngoscopy versus direct laryngoscopy for adult patients requiring tracheal intubation. In: Lewis SR, editor. Cochrane Database of Systematic Reviews [Internet]. Chichester, UK: John Wiley & Sons, Ltd; 2016 [cited 2017 Aug 8]. p. CD011136. Available from: http://www.ncbi.nlm.nih.gov/pubmed/27844477

[135] Cook TM, Astin JP, Kelly FE. Airway Management in ICU: Three Years on from NAP4. ICU. 2014;**142**(2). Matrix (https://goo.gl/a8wKhi)

[136] Wetsch WA, Carlitscheck M, Spelten O, Teschendorf P, Hellmich M, Genzwurker H V, et al. Success rates and endotracheal tube insertion times of experienced emergency physicians using five video laryngoscopes: A randomised trial in a simulated trapped car accident victim. European Journal of Anaesthesiology [Internet]. 2011;**28**(12):849-858. Available from: http://www.ncbi.nlm.nih.gov/pubmed/21986981

[137] Martínez-Hurtado E, Lucena de Pablo E, Sanchez Merchante M, De Luis Cabezón N. Videolaryngoscopy data record. A reality that is possible. In: Conference: World Airway Management Meeting Website—WAMM2015, At Dublin [Internet]. 2015. Available from: https://www.researchgate.net/publication/283720966_Videolaryngoscopy_Data_Record_A_Reality_That_Is_Possible

Chapter 3

# Endotracheal Intubation in Children: Practice Recommendations, Insights, and Future Directions

Maribel Ibarra-Sarlat, Eduardo Terrones-Vargas,
Lizett Romero-Espinoza,
Graciela Castañeda-Muciño,
Alejandro Herrera-Landero and
Juan Carlos Núñez-Enríquez

Additional information is available at the end of the chapter

http://dx.doi.org/10.5772/intechopen.70356

**Abstract**

Management of airway is mandatory in a critically ill child with severe trauma or any other situation that threatens his or her life. It is important, that clinicians who attend critically ill pediatric patients requiring airway management know the rapid sequence intubation (RSI) procedure, identify a patient with difficult airway, know the devices and techniques for the management of difficult airway, and look for receiving a formal training in endotracheal intubation (ETI). Future strategies for teaching and/or training clinicians in pediatric and neonatal ETI should be evaluated through conducting controlled clinical trials to identify which type will be the most effective by considering the less number of attempts and complications.

**Keywords:** endotracheal intubation, children, review, training, procedure

## 1. Introduction

Management and securing permeability of airway are mandatory in a critically ill child with severe trauma or any other situation that threatens his or her life. Airway's management can be defined as the performance of maneuvers and the use of devices that enable a correct and safe ventilation to patients that need this care.

Endotracheal intubation (ETI) is one of the procedures that every physician attending critically ill pediatric patients must not only know but also getting the skills and experience necessaries to effectively perform.

In this chapter, we will summarize the most practical recommendations of ETI technique in children. In addition, we will discuss important anatomical particularities of the children's airway. We include a section of devices that could help permeate the airway of pediatric patients with a difficult airway; and recent results of studies conducted regarding the association between the level of previous training in pediatric ETI and success rates.

**1.1. Indications of ETI in children**

1. Patient with an unstable airway. In this category, integrity of airway is affected by different infectious, anatomical and neurological diseases. Some examples are: (a) upper airway infectious (CROUP, bacterial tracheitis, etc.), (b) traumatisms, (c) congenital syndromes accompanied with macroglossia or micrognathia, (d) cystic hygroma, (e) branchial cleft cyst, (f) thyroglossal duct cyst, and (g) those patients with a large anterior mediastinal mass (non-Hodgkin lymphoma, acute leukemia, etc.). During childhood, the most common cause is infections [1].

2. Patient with neurological dysfunction secondary to trauma, seizures, metabolic disease, or toxic ingestion. Classically, we can find patients with a Glasgow Coma Scale (GCS) score of 8 or less, or a deterioration in the GCS score from 14 to 10.

3. Patient with impaired gas exchange:

    a. Hypoxia. One of the most common indications of ETI. Clinically, the patient presents with respiratory distress, tachypnea, increased work of breathing, and an increase in alveolar-arterial gradient. Some causes of hypoxia are airway obstruction, hypoventilation, ventilation/perfusion mismatch, hemoglobinopathies, abnormal pulmonary diffusion, and intracardiac right to left shunt.

    b. Hypercarbia. The pathophysiologic phenomenon consists of alteration in ventilation. There exists a reduced lung compliance and a V/Q mismatch increasing physiologic dead space. Alteration in ventilation can also be secondary to muscle weakness, altered mental status, exposure to toxins, or iatrogenic oversedation.

4. Patient with lower airway obstruction. Hypercarbia, tachypnea, increased work of breathing, wheezing, and a prolonged expiratory phase are characteristic. As lower obstruction progresses, dynamic hyperinflation and air trapping worsen, leading to a silent chest (inaudible breath sounds). This obstruction is common in asthma and bronchiolitis. We must remember that children can get intubated by this indication but it has been described an increase in mean airway pressure that may impede venous return. Therefore, under this indication children should only be intubated in EXTREME CIRCUMSTANCES [1].

5. Patient with a reduction of mechanical load, as seen in shock state and some patients with cardiovascular dysfunction.

## 2. Practice recommendations for pediatric endotracheal intubation

### 2.1. Rapid sequence intubation

By using rapid sequence intubation (RSI) method, a clinician can effectively achieve pediatric endotracheal intubation (ETI), however, we previously must identify if the patient has one or more of the following features related with a difficult airway [2]:

- To have congenital abnormalities related with a difficult airway such as Pierre Robins Syndrome and/or Treacher Collins Syndrome.
- A previous difficult ETI.
- A poor mouth opening, large tongue or tonsils, small chin, short mandible, decreased neck mobility, and/or an evidence of partial upper airway obstruction.

Note: later in this chapter, you can find information about the causes, techniques, and a variety of devices a clinician may use for the management of children with difficult airway.

#### *2.1.1. Preparation*

1. If it is not performed in an emergency setting (elective intubation), an informed consent must be obtained from the child's parents explaining the technique, complications, and benefits of performing the procedure [3].
2. All the materials to be used should be functional.
3. Team should consist of three persons (at least).
4. Patient's heart and respiratory rate, blood pressure, oxygen saturation, (capnography when available) must be monitored during the procedure.
5. Oxygen supply must be at least 10 l/min and suction equipment must be available and it must have pressures around 80–120 mm Hg.

*Equipment*

1. An appropriate mask and bag for ventilation. We must select the mask size that fits the nasal bridge and the chin of the patient without covering the eyes (**Figure 1**). Bag used for infants and young children is named pediatric bag (which provides a tidal volume of approximately 400–500 ml); for older children and adolescents, an adult bag should be used (providing a tidal volume of 1000 ml) [3–5].
2. Endotracheal tubes (ETs). Uncuffed ETs are mainly indicated for neonates, infants, and young children (<8 years). The correct size of these ETs can be calculated according to the equation (child's age/4) + 4. On the other hand, the formula (child's age/2) + 3.5 might be used for cuffed ETs. Other methods to calculate ETs size include comparing the child's fifth finger with the internal diameter of the ET or by using resuscitation tape such as the Broselow Luten tape, and it is recommendable to have one size larger and smaller of the selected tube.
3. Stylet. Adult sized for 5.5 tubes and beyond, pediatric ones for lower endotracheal tubes.

4. Laryngoscope handle and blade. The first one can be an adult or pediatric one, and the second can be straight or curved depending on the experience of the laryngoscopist. The blades used in pediatrics ranged from 00 (extremely premature neonates) to 4. Blades 0–1 are used for preterm and full-term neonates, size 1 for infants. At age 2, size 2 blade; at this age, a curved blade can be used. For ages 10 and above, a number 3 blade is recommended.
5. Colorimetric end tidal carbon dioxide devices or capnography monitors.
6. Tape or a commercial holder to secure the endotracheal tube.
7. Syringe for cuff inflation.
8. Nasogastric and orogastric tubes.

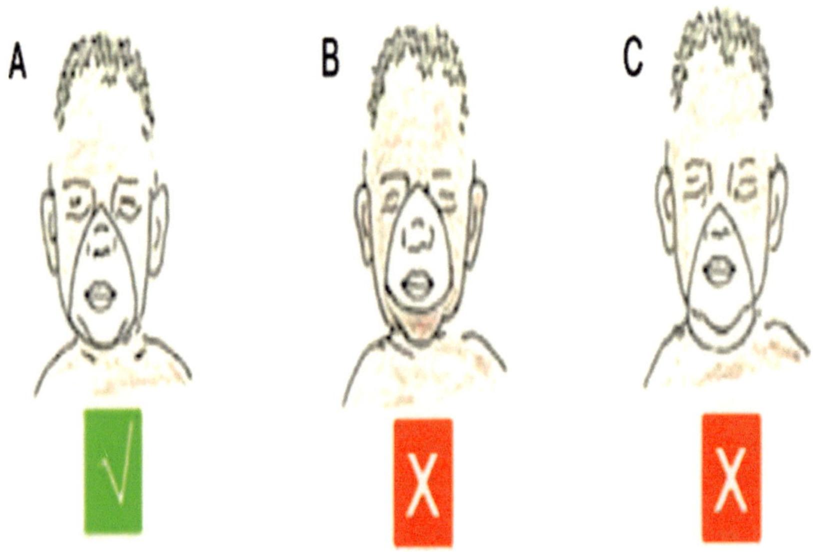


**Figure 1.** (A) The correct size for the child because it covers the area between nasal bridge and chin. (B) The mask elected is not correct, it covers part of the eyes of the patient. (C) The mask elected is not correct it covers the area far from the chin.

---

**Tips and tricks**

**To remember all the preparatory equipment before starting intubation**

You can use the **STOP MAID** mnemonic to remember all the preparatory equipment before starting ETI procedure:

Suction;

Tools for intubation;

Oxygen;

Positioning (sniffing position so that the external auditory canal is anterior to shoulder);

Monitors;

Assistant, Ambu bag with facemask, airway devices;

Intravenous access;

Drugs (sedation, neuromuscular blocking medications).

### 2.1.2. Preoxygenation phase

With all the necessary tools already prepared, next, we must position the patient for the denominated preoxygenation phase. This position consists in a sniffing situation avoiding hyperextension and/or hyperflexion of the neck. The correct sniffing position is the one with exterior auditory canal anterior to the shoulders (**Figure 2**).

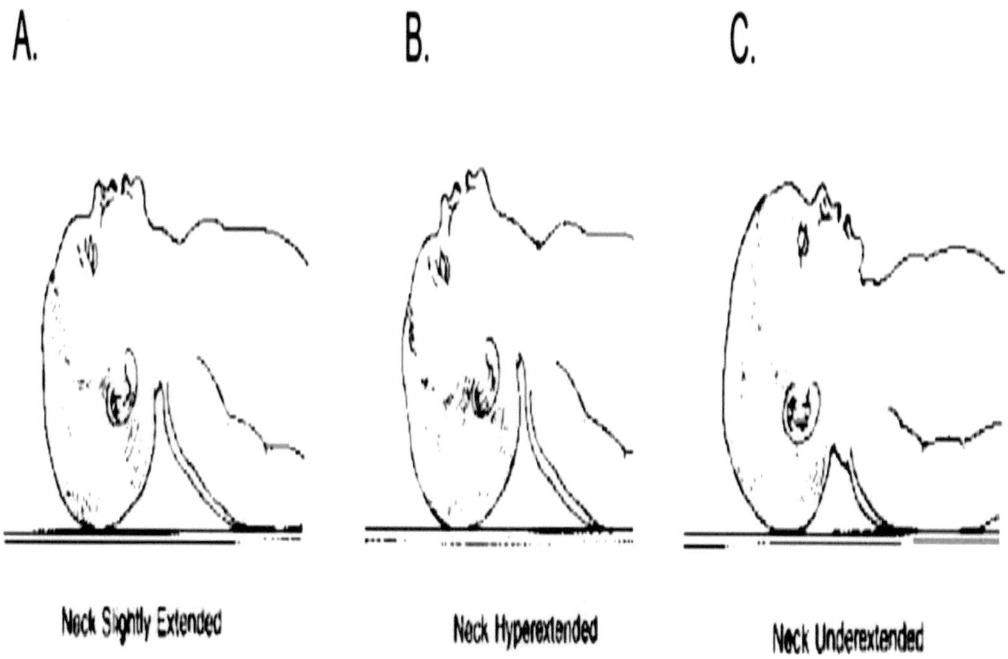


**Figure 2.** (A) Correct sniffing position is shown the external auditory canal is anterior to the shoulders of the patient. (B) Incorrect position because neck is hyperextended. (C) Incorrect position because patient's neck has hyperflexion.

Selection of ventilation technique relies on the number of persons available at preoxygenation phase:

- One-person ventilation technique. The head must be positioned backwards, using the C-E technique and the chin must be elevated pressing and sealing the mask to the face. Sealing is very important. We may corroborate that ventilation technique is correct when elevation of the chest is observed (**Figure 3**).
- Two-person ventilation technique. One member of the health care professional team will use the C-E technique but now with two hands while the other person will be pressing the bag (**Figure 4**).

After patient is positioned, then, ventilation must start with 100% inspired oxygen creating an oxygen reservoir. It is important to avoid hyperventilation. Therefore, a slow ventilation lasting around a second each must be applied being overall preoxygenation phase duration 3–5 min.

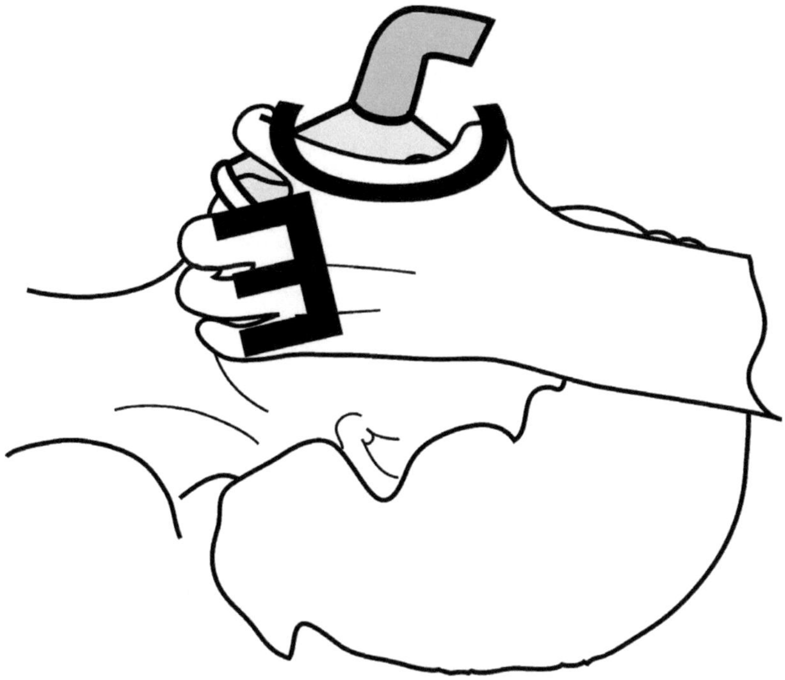

**Figure 3.** One-person C-E ventilation technique is illustrated.

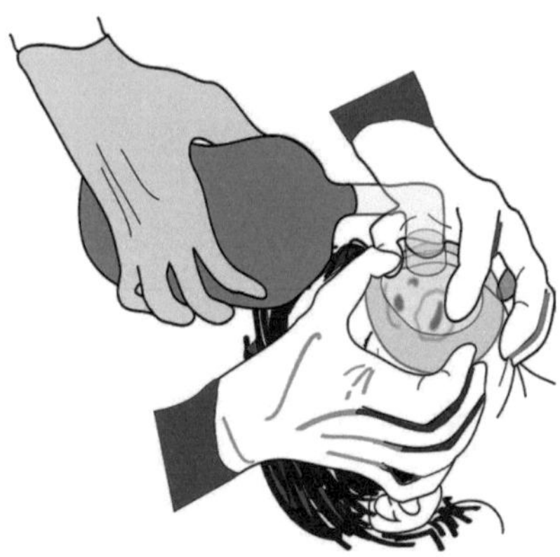

**Figure 4.** Two-person C-E ventilation technique. First person is doing a double hand C-E maneuver while a second person (not shown in the image) is pressing the bag.

### *2.1.3. Sedation and neuromuscular blockade*

Premedication increases success rate of pediatric ETI independently from degree of previous training [6]. By using the rapid sequence intubation in children, success rate of 52% and a complication rate of 61% can be achieved [7], however, sedation can be omitted in obtunded or comatose patients and neuromuscular blockade must be avoided in patients with difficult airway. **Table 1** summarizes the drugs, indications, and doses used for sedation and neuromuscular blockade during pediatric ETI procedure.

http://dx.doi.org/10.5772/intechopen.70356

| Medications | | Indications | Doses (IV) |
|---|---|---|---|
| Sedation | Etomidate | Hemodynamic instability, neuroprotective | 0.3 mg/kg |
| | Ketamine | Hemodynamic instability, patients with bronchospasm and septic shock | 1–2 mg/kg |
| | Midazolam | It can cause hemodynamic instability | 0.2–0.3 mg/kg |
| | Propofol | In hemodynamically stable patients | 1–1.5 mg/kg |
| | Thiopental | Neuroprotection | 3–5 mg/kg |
| NM blockers | Rocuronium | For children in which succinylcholine is contraindicated | 0.6–1.2 mg/kg |
| | Succinylcholine | Do not use in extensive crush injury, chronic myopathy | 2 mg/kg |

**Table 1.** Drugs, indications, doses for achieving sedation and neuromuscular (NM) blockade during pediatric ETI.

### *2.1.4. Procedure*

Clinician may most easily perform direct laryngoscopy by standing behind to the patient's head and with height of the bed adjusted to the level of the laryngoscopist xiphoid appendix (**Figure 5**). After sedation and neuromuscular blocking, the clinician must perform a scissor maneuver to open mouth before laryngoscopy. Then, laryngoscope must be held in the left hand (regardless of dominance), inserting the blade in the right side of the patient's mouth along the base of the tongue following the contour of the pharynx, and sweeping the tongue to the left.

Once the tongue and soft tissues are retracted, clinician must recognize the following anatomic structures: epiglottis, arytenoid cartilage, and esophagus (**Figure 6**). After identifying epiglottis, this must be elevated exposing the vocal cords by handling laryngoscope at a 45° angle. Next step, endotracheal tube (ET) must be inserted into the trachea by holding it (with right hand) like a pencil (**Figure 7**).

ET insertion in airway must be confirmed by the observation chest wall rise and down with ventilations, auscultation of breath sounds in both axillae and not heard over stomach, and, to observe an adequate oxygen saturation (>90%). Radiographically, a correct position of the

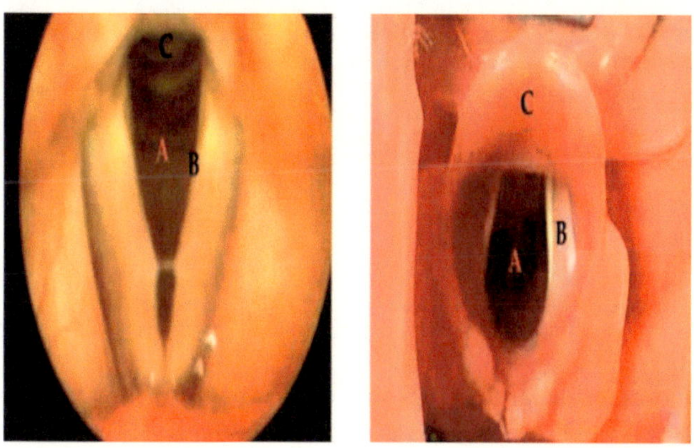


**Figure 5.** Proper position of laryngoscopist and correct introduction of laryngoscope after opening patient's mouth through a scissor maneuver (not shown).

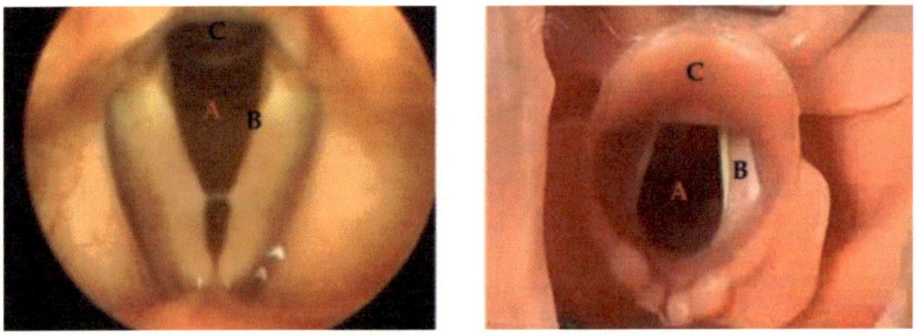


**Figure 6.** A comparison between a real larynx and a model. Structures of the larynx must be identified before trying to insert ET. (A) Glottis, (B) Vocal cords. (C) Epiglottis.

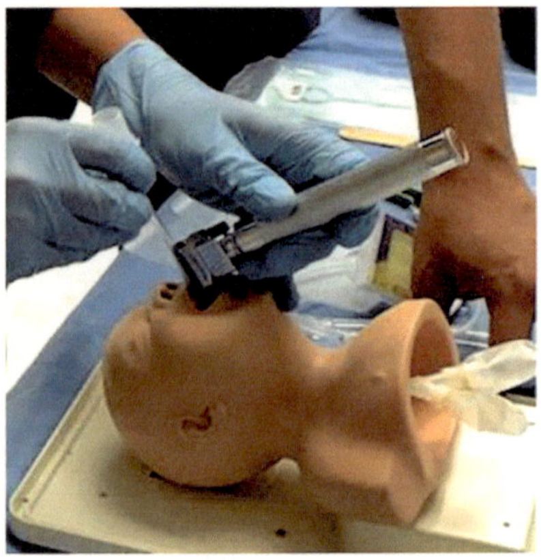

**Figure 7.** ET is introduced like a pencil into the airway.

**Tips and tricks**

**To identify epiglottis and/or glottic structures**

If epiglottis and/or glottic structures are not visible, blade must be pulled back slowly until they are visible. Other useful technique for helping to identify epiglottis and/or glottic structures is the named "Sellick maneuver" or so known as "cricoid pressure" (**Figure 8**). To perform it, another member of the reanimation team slightly push the region of cricoid cartilage while laryngoscopist observes the structures and introduce ET.

**To calculate ETT length insertion**

ET length insertion can be determined by any of the following two formulas [5, 8, 9]:

#1- (Patient's age (in years)/2) + 12

#2- ET internal diameter * 3

Note: we recommend first equation because it has been reported as more accurate.

tube is below the thoracic inlet and 3 cm above the carina (**Figure 9**). In case of ETT is located at esophagus or right bronchus, immediate measures must be taken to remove it and secure an adequate ventilation of patient (**Figures 9** and **10**).

http://dx.doi.org/10.5772/intechopen.70356

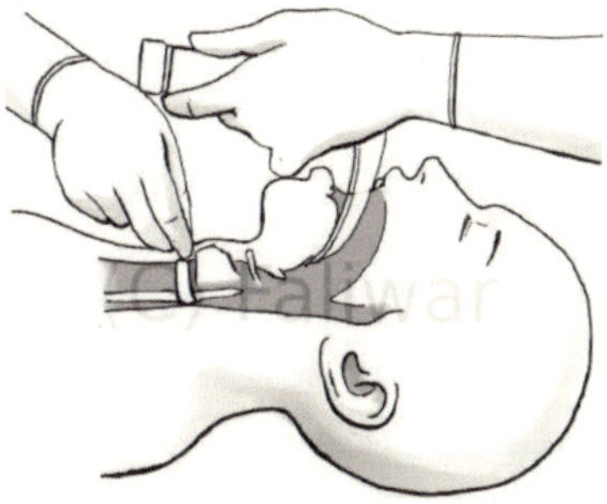

**Figure 8.** Sellick's Maneuver (also known as cricoid pressure).

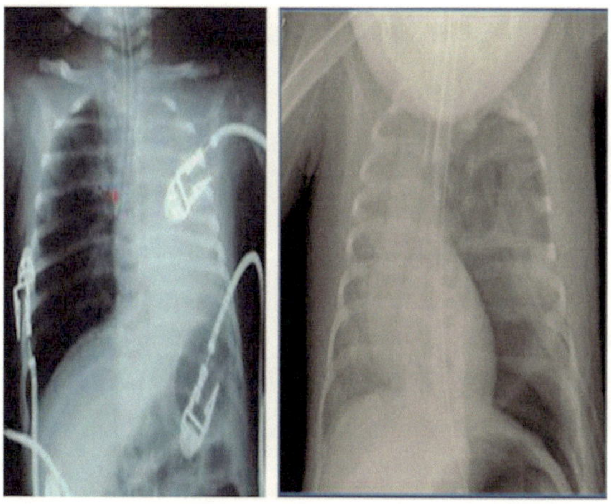

**Figure 9.** X-ray on the left shows a misplaced endotracheal tube which is in the right bronchus. Right X-ray shows a correct placement of the endotracheal tube, where the tip is located above the carina.

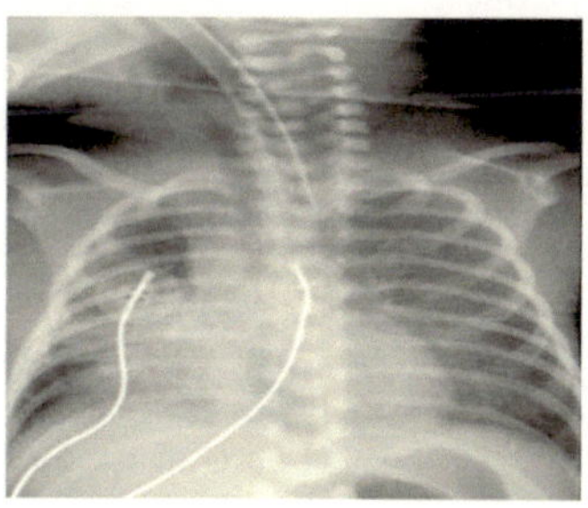

**Figure 10.** ET located in esophagus.

Tips and tricks [5, 10]

**In case of acute respiratory deterioration after intubation**

**Remember the mnemonic DONE** which can help you to identify the probable causes:

**Deviation** of ETT to the main bronchus or misplacement during suction. Signs that can suggest this are asymmetric elevation of the thorax or asymmetric auscultation, specially the right hemithorax.

**Obstruction** due to secretions obstructing tube's lumen.

**Pneumothorax** if are present signs as breath sounds diminished on the affected side, conduction of vocal vibrations to the surface of the chest may be increased, and hyperresonant at percussion.

**Equipment**, if problem is in the ventilator hardware or software.

## 3. Neonatal intubation

### 3.1. Indications

ETI in neonates can be most commonly performed as an emergency procedure or as part of an elective or semi-elective treatment:

1. Emergency. When mask ventilation or non-invasive mechanical ventilation fails, in case of structural or congenital airway abnormalities, diaphragmatic hernia, prolonged cardiopulmonary resuscitation, if thoracic compressions are needed, surfactant administration and for direct tracheal aspirations if thick secretions exist [11].
2. Elective/semi elective. Prematurity, positive pressure ventilation lasting more than 1-min, in case of ET must be changed, and in patients with an unstable airway [11].

### 3.2. Important anatomical considerations in neonates

In comparison to older children, adolescents and adults, anatomy of neonatal upper airway structures is different, being neonates a subpopulation where the ETI becomes a challenge. Some of these differences are the following: (a) a tongue proportionately larger, in consequence, trying to sweep it during ETI might be difficult and its backward movement might result in an airway obstruction; (b) epiglottis is longer, narrower, less flexible, and sometimes omega-shaped; (c) a cranial position of larynx can be an obstacle for observing the glottis during laryngoscopy, being this issue the reason why is preferable to use straight blades rather than curved ones in neonates; and (d) trachea is proportionally shorter and narrower [12, 13].

It is important to highlight, that neonates <1000 g, >4000 g, or those with congenital craniofacial abnormalities have less chance to be intubated at first attempt, representing a subgroup of neonates with a difficult airway which require special attention [14].

http://dx.doi.org/10.5772/intechopen.70356

On the other hand, each attempt of intubation in neonates provokes injury of the mucosa which subsequently leads to an inflammation decreasing the caliber of the field of observation, and therefore, making the intubation less effective. Currently, it has been recommended a limit of 20 s for each intubation attempt in neonates, and if it fails, the ET must be removed and patient must be ventilated with a mask-bag reservoir until recovery [11, 15, 16].

| Tips and tricks |
|---|
| **Premedication phase in neonates is different from older children** |
| In neonates, premedication phase must be only used as part of an elective ETI and not for emergency situations. |
| The American Academy of Pediatrics (AAP) and the Canadian Pediatric Society (CPS) recommend a combination of vagolytic agents and neuromuscular blockers for premedication phase in neonates. Also, the AAP recommends that muscular blockers and sedatives must not be used alone without analgesia [3]. |

| Tips and tricks |
|---|
| **ET size election for neonates** |
| Election of ET size based on neonate's weight and gestational age: |

| Weight (g) | Gestational age (weeks) | ET size (internal diameter in mm) |
|---|---|---|
| <1000 | <28 | 2.5 |
| 1000–2000 | 28–34 | 3.0 |
| >2000 | >34 | 3.4 |

### 3.3. Estimating length insertion of ET in neonates

Two methods may be used, and the objective is to place the tip of ET in the middle portion of trachea.

**a.** DNT method

We must add 1 cm to the distance (cm) between the newborn's nasal septum and ear tragus (**Figure 11**) [17].

**b.** Gestational age method (**Table 2**)

**c.** "7-8-9 rule" method: in 1979, Tochen described a simple equation for the ET insertion length based on patient's weight at birth.

Formula: 1.17 * weight at birth (kg) + 5.58.

This equation has been supported by the AAP and the American Heart Association (AHA), establishing ET insertion length can be calculated by adding 6 cm to the newborn weight (e.g., for a newborn weighing 1 kg = 1 + 6 = 7 cm), from the patient's lip [14].

**Tips and tricks**

**ET length insertion when nasotracheal intubation is used**

When nasotracheal intubation is performed, the ET length must increase in 20% (e.g., for a newborn weighing 2 kg: (2 kg + 6) × 1.2 = 9.6 cm). We must also take in consideration that the 7-8-9 rule can overestimate the insertion length in newborns with a birth weight less than 1000 g. In consequence, it is preferred to use the gestational age method (**Table 2**) [18].

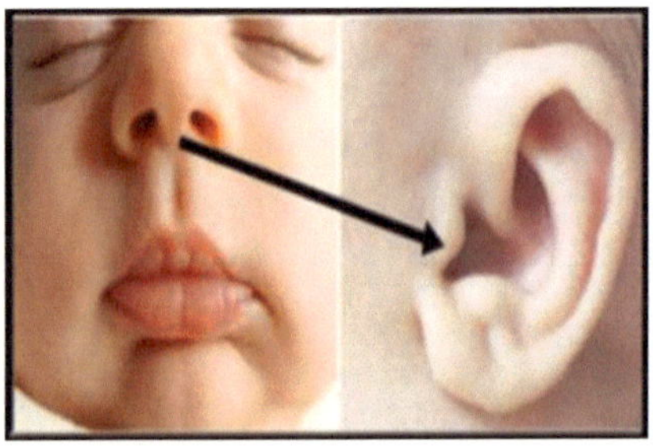

**Figure 11.** DNT method.

| Gestational age (weeks) | ET length insertion (cm) from the patient's lips | Weight (g) |
|---|---|---|
| 23–24 | 5.5 | 500–600 |
| 25–26 | 6.0 | 700–800 |
| 27–29 | 6.5 | 900–1000 |
| 30–32 | 7.0 | 1100–1400 |
| 33–34 | 7.5 | 1500–1800 |
| 35–37 | 8.0 | 1900–2400 |
| 38–40 | 8.5 | 2500–3100 |
| 41–43 | 9.0 | 3200–4200 |

**Table 2.** Gestational age method to calculate ET length insertion [18].

## 4. Management of the child with difficult airway (DA)

Difficult airway can be defined as the clinical situation in which a conventionally trained physician has trouble for achieving an effective upper airway ventilation with a face mask, for tracheal intubation or both and where interact patient's factors, setting conditions and operator skills [19]. First, we must evaluate child's airway to identify those clinical, and/or laboratory factors that could make difficult to achieve ETI. Among the anatomical factors related with DA are the form and size of mouth, nose, mandible, neck, existence of masses or congenital malformations, and other childhood diseases that eventually could difficult ETI (**Figure 12**, **Tables 3** and **4**) [20–24].

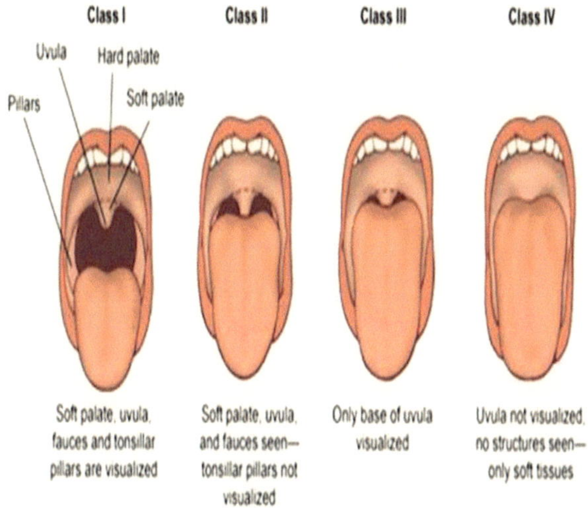


**Figure 12.** Difficult airway for ETI based on modified Mallampati classification [25, 26].

- Cranium's bone displacement. Apert syndrome, Crouzon syndrome, hydrocephalus
- Mandible hypoplasia. Pierre Robin syndrome, Treacher Collins syndrome, Goldenhar syndrome, Apert syndrome
- Abnormal neck mobility. Klippel-Fleil syndrome, Down syndrome, mucopolisacaridosis
- Limited oral aperture: Sheldon Freedman syndrome, Hallerman-Strieff syndrome, bullous epidermolysis
- Small oral cavity: Pierre Robin syndrome, Treacher-Collins syndrome
- Macroglossia: hypothyroidism, Beckwith Wiedemann syndrome, Down syndrome, mucopolisacaridosis
- Airway or neck masses: cystic hygroma, teratomas, hemangiomas
- Laryngeal or subglottic anomalies

**Table 3.** Pediatric syndromes associated with DA.

### 4.1. Devices and techniques for the management of the child with DA

DA devices can be classified according to the anatomical structure from where they will act and/or on their optical properties [27]:

### 4.2. Supraglottic airway devices

#### *4.2.1. Classic laryngeal mask*

It was developed in 1980 by Dr Archie Brain and forms part of the rescue devices in the ASA algorithm for the difficult airway management. It was designed to be situated in the

| Infectious | Traumatic | Neoplastic | Inflammatory | Neurologic | Other |
|---|---|---|---|---|---|
| • Epiglottitis<br>• Abscess (submandibular, retropharyngeal, Ludwig's angina)<br>• Croup<br>• Papillomatosis | • Foreign body<br>• Cervical column lesion<br>• Skull base fracture<br>• Maxillary or mandible lesion<br>• Laryngeal fracture<br>• Postintubation laryngeal edema<br>• Facial trauma<br>• Burns | • Upper airway tumors (pharynx, larynx)<br>• Inferior airway tumors (trachea, bronchi, mediastinal)<br>• Post-radiation area | • Angioedema<br>• Anaphylactic shock (laryngeal edema)<br>• Anquilosis<br>• Juvenile Rheumatoid arthritis | • Spastic cerebral paralysis<br>• Tetanus | • Lung hemorrhage<br>• Obesity<br>• Cranium-facial malformations<br>• Micrognathia<br>• Superior incisive protrusion<br>• Short and wide neck<br>• Big tongue<br>• Previous intubation difficulty<br>• Oral aperture limitation<br>• Clift lip and palate<br>• Mallampati classes 3 or 4 (**Figure 12**) |

**Table 4.** Childhood diseases associated with DA.

hypopharynx, with an anterior aperture situated at the glottis entrance, the mask's border is made of a silicone inflatable cuff, sealing the hypopharynx permitting positive pressure ventilation (less than 20 cm $H_2O$). The mask is introduced using the index finger of the dominant hand as a guide towards the hypopharynx, following the palate's curvature, until a resistance is felt, then the cuff must be inflated with a determined volume (the specific volume comes in a legend on the mask itself and depends of the number of the mask). Choosing the size mask depends on the weight of the patient. As complications of the procedure we can find aspiration of gastric contents, uvula, and pharyngeal pillars lesions (**Figure 13**).

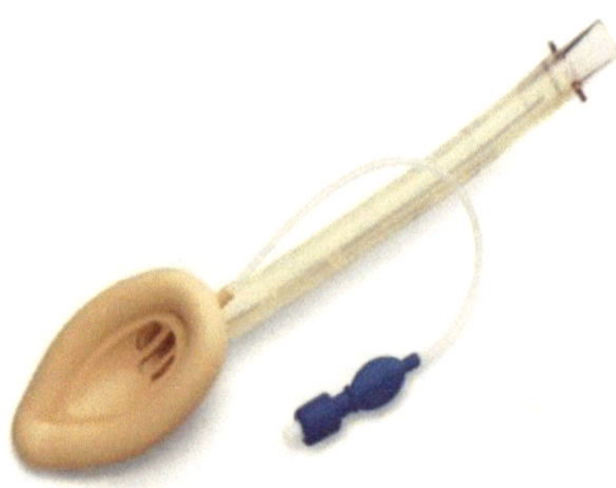

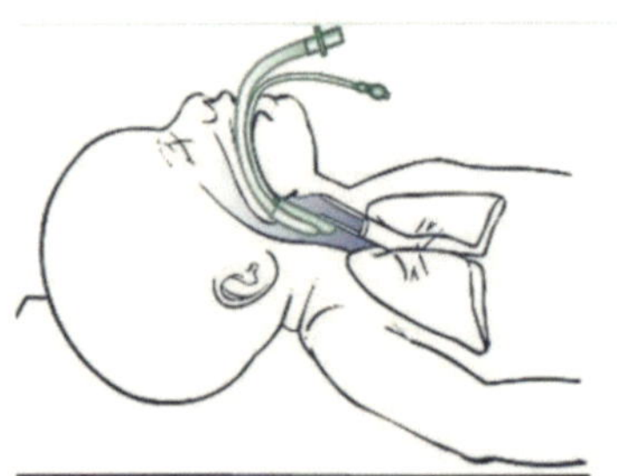

**Figure 13.** Laryngeal mask.

#### *4.2.2. ProSeal laryngeal mask airway*

In 2000 Brain published the description of a new laryngeal mask that tried to improve the airway's protection against gastric aspiration. This was accomplished by including a second tube lateral to the airway's tube and which in its distal end is located on the tip of the mask. This tube has the function of separating the digestive tract from the respiratory, and also Permits accessing the stomach with an orogastric probe (**Figure 14**) [28].

#### *4.2.3. Fastrach or intubation laryngeal mask (ILMA)*

This type of laryngeal mask is designed with the objective of achieving intubation through the mask itself, it consists of an anatomically curved rigid tube, wide enough to accept in it endotracheal tubes this end is united to rigid metal loop that makes the insertion much easier, removal, and adjustment of the position with one hand only. Once installed, and ventilation achieved an ET is inserted, the mask is then removed maintaining the tube in place, with a specially designed stylet, so that after the mask is removed the ET remains in place (**Figure 15**).

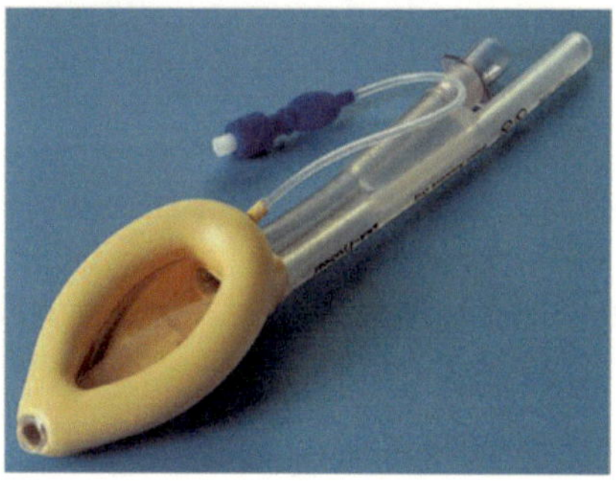

**Figure 14.** ProSeal laryngeal mask airway.

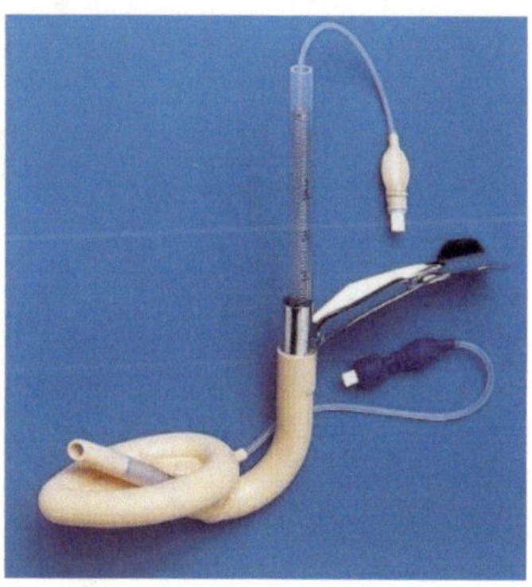

**Figure 15.** FASTRACH or intubation laryngeal mask (ILMA).

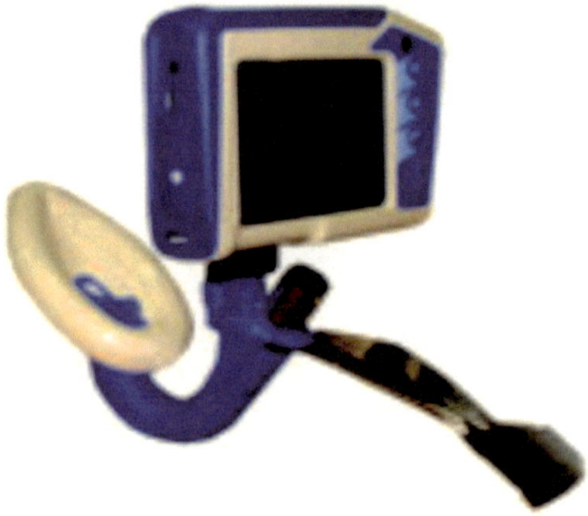

**Figure 16.** New type of Fastrach laryngeal mask.

Other type of *Fastrach laryngeal mask* (*2005*) *with an incorporated camera,* permits once it has been introduced into the hypopharynx, setting a monitor on the outer part of the mask so that it can be possible introducing an ET under direct vision (**Figure 16**).

*4.2.4. Combitube*

This device can only be used to ventilate in emergency situations. It was designed in Austria in the year 1980. Insertion is easy for any person and insertion is blindfold. It consists of a double lumen latex tube that combines the functions of an esophageal obturator and a conventional ET. Combitube has two balloons which inflate from the exterior. First one corresponds to an oropharyngeal balloon (85–100 ml of capacity) situated in a proximal position to the pharyngeal perforations with a function of serves as a sealing of the oral and nasal cavity; second one, is called traqueo-esophagic balloon, and needs a volume of 12–15 ml to seal the trachea or esophagus. Combitube can be placed either in the esophagus or in trachea, and in case of tube passes to the esophagus, the patient can still be ventilated because the perforations existing in combitube esophageal lumen, and the stomach can be aspirated from the tracheal lumen. In case of combitube is set in the trachea, the patient can also be ventilated from the trachea lumen (**Figure 17**) [29, 30].

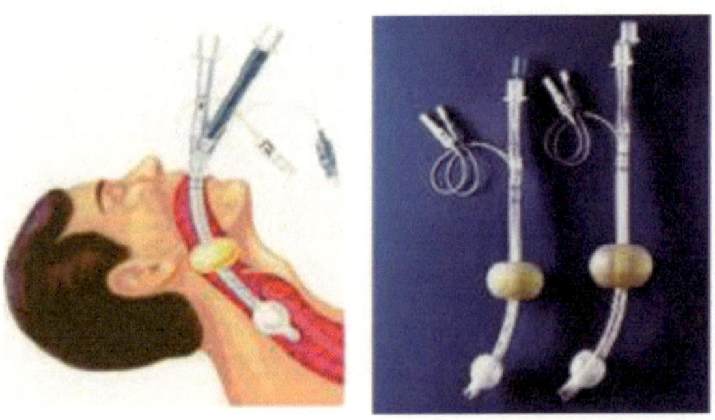

**Figure 17.** Combitube.

### 4.3. Transglottic airway devices

#### 4.3.1. Gum Elastic Bougie

*Eschman Guide* or *Gum Elastic Bougie* (*GEB*) is a semi-flexible guide of polyester covered in resin (to avoid laryngeal trauma). GEB has a 15-Fr diameter and can be introduced in 6 mm internal diameter tubes. Insertion technique consists of sliding the angulated tip underneath the epiglottis, then, dragging at the tracheal cartilages must be perceived (**Figure 18**) [31].

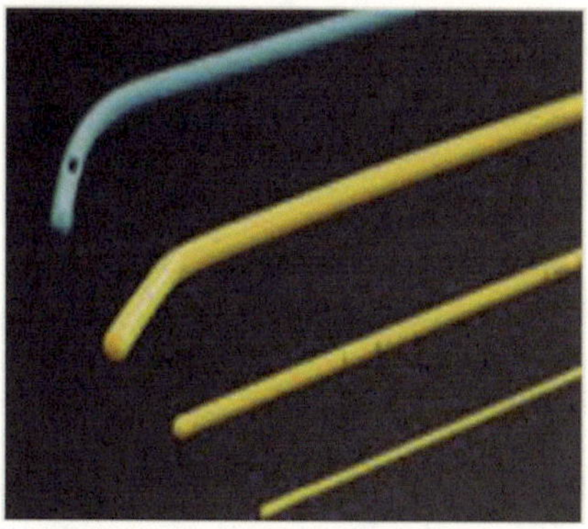

**Figure 18.** Gum Elastic Bougie (GEB).

#### 4.3.2. Lightwand device (Trachlight)

In some countries, a lighted stylet is used for ETI, this is the called *Trachlight*. It is based on transillumination of the soft tissue of the neck with a high effectivity for achieving intubation in an approximate time of 25 s (**Figure 19**) [32].

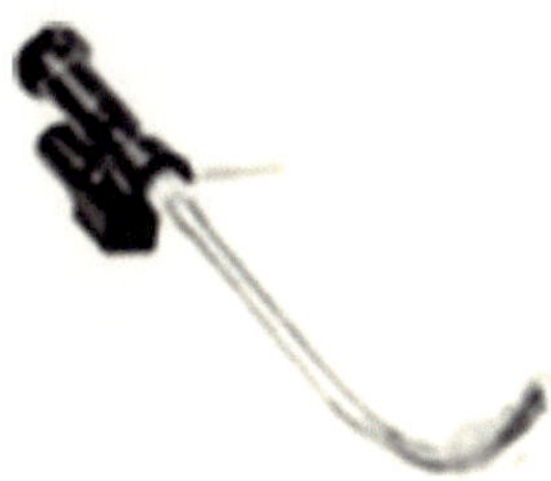

**Figure 19.** Lightwand device (Trachlight).

### 4.4. Optical devices

#### 4.4.1. Video laryngoscopes

They are laryngoscopes that carry in its distal blade's end a high-resolution video camera to visualize the glottis and to introduce an ET without the need of observing the glottis directly but through a high-resolution screen which can be located in the same device or at the patient's side. Among the main complications reported are the soft palate lesions (**Figure 20**).

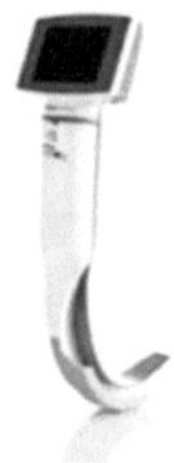

**Figure 20.** Video laryngoscope.

## 5. Insights and future directions

### 5.1. Direct laryngoscopy vs. video laryngoscopy

Learning curve (LC) in the case of the direct laryngoscopy requires of approximately of 45–50 previous intubations [33], while LC for video laryngoscopy is around 5 attempts. ETI using a video laryngoscopy is possible with little training, due to transmitted image from the blade's distal tip makes easier the visualization of the larynx entrance. When intubation attempts using Miller or Macintosh laryngoscopes or video laryngoscopy fail other methods to secure pediatric airway are recommended to be used (i.e. supraglottic devices). Recent studies have reported that ETI with video laryngoscopy even performed by less experienced medical personnel, increases significantly the success rate in the first attempt in comparison with direct laryngoscopy [34]; moreover, it has been reported that video laryngoscopy decreases the intubation time with less desaturation and less failure rate when it is compared with conventional laryngoscopy [35, 36]. Nevertheless, other video laryngoscope methods (GlideScope) implying other type of learning (mainly based on exploration), have resulted to be inferior to direct laryngoscopy regarding the time required for ETI [37].

### 5.2. Importance of formal training in pediatric ETI

Until date there is no standard definition for the term proficiency in pediatric/neonatal airway ETI. In a recent study, defined a formal training in pediatric airway management as having received at least 2 weeks of training by pediatric anesthesiology teachers. In that study was reported that after formal training, intubation success rate increased from 65.1 to 75.7% ($p = 0.01$), and it was observed a significant decreasing in the number of intubation attempts ($p = 0.01$). However, they did not find statistically significant differences in the time for achieving Intubation nor for the frequency of complications [38].

In a study conducted by Kerrey et al., where rapid sequence intubation technique was used, pediatricians in emergency departments and anesthesiologist had higher success rates (88–91%) in comparison to physicians in formation (45%) [7]. These results were similar to the reported by Goto et al. where intubation success was higher at the first attempt in pediatricians (OR 2.36; CI 95% 1.11–4.97) and in emergency room physicians (OR 3.2; CI 95% 1.78–5.83) in comparison to pediatric residents of the first and second year [39].

It has also been evaluated the skills for neonatal ETI between residents. Interestingly, skills significantly improved with a success rate from 27% during the first year of formation to 79% for the second year. Number of attempts also improved decreasing from 3.6 to 1.2 from the first to the second year, respectively [38]. This and other study results highlight the relevance of implementing training strategies from early stages of education in medicine to effectively achieve ETI in children with the less number of attempts and complications [6, 40, 41].

#### *5.2.1. ETI training models, live models, and simulation training sessions for increasing success in pediatric and neonatal intubation*

Recently, it has been mentioned that there are no differences in the learning curve or the skills for performing neonatal intubation by comparing live models versus ETI training models. Retention curves with a follow-up of 6, 18 and 52 weeks remain constant after 6 weeks and get lost after 18 and 52 weeks; although, retention is higher when skill levels are higher too [42, 43]. Additionally, it has been reported that educational interventions such as training sessions using didactic and simulation components have not been related with an improvement in intubation success rate; even, performance points decrease after 8 weeks of the intervention [44]. Importantly, other studies have not found differences in pediatric ETI success rate at first attempt by comparing groups with and without training [45].

## 6. Conclusions

It is important to highlight, that clinicians who attend critically ill pediatric patients requiring airway management know the rapid sequence intubation procedure, identify a patient with difficult airway, know the devices and techniques for the management of difficult airway, and look for receiving a formal training. Future strategies for teaching and/or training clinicians in pediatric and neonatal ETI should be evaluated through conducting controlled clinical trials to identify which type is the most effective by considering the less number of attempts and complications.

## Author details

Maribel Ibarra-Sarlat[1], Eduardo Terrones-Vargas[2], Lizett Romero-Espinoza[3], Graciela Castañeda-Muciño[1], Alejandro Herrera-Landero[4] and Juan Carlos Núñez-Enríquez[1]*

*Address all correspondence to: jcarlos_nu@hotmail.com

1 UMAE Hospital de Pediatría Centro Médico Nacional Siglo XXI, Instituto Mexicano del Seguro Social, México City, Mexico

2 Unidad de Cuidados Intensivos Pediátricos, Hospital Infantil de México Federico Gómez, Secretaria de Salud, México City, Mexico

3 UMAE Hospital Gineco-Obstetricia No.3 "Dr. Victor Manuel Espinosa De Los Reyes Sánchez", Centro Médico Nacional La Raza, Mexico City, Mexico

4 Hospital de Traumatología y Ortopedia «Lomas Verdes», Instituto Mexicano del Seguro Social, State of Mexico, Mexico

## References

[1] Rimensberger P. Pediatric and Neonatal Mechanical Ventilation. From Basics to Clinical Practice. 1st ed. New Delhi, India: Springer-Verlag Berlin Heidelberg; 2015. 1642 p

[2] Russo SG, Becke K. Expected difficult airway in children. Current Opinion in Anaesthesiology. 2015;**28**(3):321-326

[3] Emergency endotracheal intubation in children [database on the Internet]. UpToDate. 2015 [cited 2017-06-01]

[4] Staple L, O'Connell K. Pediatric rapid sequence intubation: An in-depth review. Pediatric Emergency Medicine Reports. 2013;**18**(1):1

[5] Kleinman ME, de Caen AR, Chameides L, Atkins DL, Berg RA, Berg MD, et al. Part 10: Pediatric basic and advanced life support: 2010 International Consensus on Cardiopulmonary Resuscitation and Emergency Cardiovascular Care Science with Treatment Recommendations. Circulation. 2010;**122**(16 Suppl 2):S466-S515

[6] Le CN, Garey DM, Leone TA, Goodmar JK, Rich W, Finer NN. Impact of premedication on neonatal intubations by pediatric and neonatal trainees. Journal of Perinatology. 2014;**34**(6):458-460

[7] Kerrey BT, Rinderknecht AS, Geis GL, Nigrovic LE, Mittiga MR. Rapid sequence intubation for pediatric emergency patients: Higher frequency of failed attempts and adverse effects found by video review. Annals of Emergency Medicine. 2012;**60**(3):251-259

[8] Curley MA, Arnold JH, Thompson JE, Fackler JC, Grant MJ, Fineman LD, et al. Clinical trial design—Effect of prone positioning on clinical outcomes in infants and children with acute respiratory distress syndrome. Journal of Critical Care. 2006;**21**(1):23-32; Discussion - 7

[9] Nichols D, Shaffner D. Rogers' Textbook of Pediatric Intensive Care. 5 ed. Philadelphia, PA: Wolters Kluwer Health; 2015

[10] Engorn B, Flerlage J. The Harriet Lane Handbook. 20 ed. Amsterdam; New York: Elsevier; 2014

[11] Weiner G, Zaichkin J. Textbook of Neonatal Resuscitation. 7 ed. Amsterdam; New York: American Academy of Pediatrics. American Heart Association; 2016

[12] Vijayasekaran S, Lioy J, Maschhoff K. Airway disorders of the fetus and neonate: An overview. Seminars in Fetal and Neonatal Medicine. 2016;**21**(4):220-229

[13] Murphy M, Walls R. Manual of Emergency Airway Management. 4 ed. Philadelphia, PA: Wolters Kluwer Health; 2012

[14] Johansen LC, Mupanemunda RH, Danha RF. Managing the newborn infant with a difficult airway. Infant. 2012;**8**(4):116-119

[15] Smereka J. Which laryngoscope method should inexperienced intubators use for child intubation? American Journal of Emergency Medicine. 2016;**34**(8):1729-1730

[16] O'Donnell CP, Kamlin CO, Davis PG, Morley CJ. Endotracheal intubation attempts during neonatal resuscitation: Success rates, duration, and adverse effects. Pediatrics. 2006;**117**(1):e16-e21

[17] Gray MM, Delaney H, Umoren R, Strandjord TP, Sawyer T. Accuracy of the nasal-tragus length measurement for correct endotracheal tube placement in a cohort of neonatal resuscitation simulators. Journal of perinatology. 2017:[Epub ahead of print]

[18] Kempley ST, Moreiras JW, Petrone FL. Endotracheal tube length for neonatal intubation. Resuscitation. 2008;**77**(3):369-373

[19] Auroy Y, Benhamou D, Pequignot F, Bovet M, Jougla E, Lienhart A. Mortality related to airway complications. Anaesthesia. 2009;**64**(4):366-370

[20] Cook TM, Woodall N, Frerk C. Major complications of airway management in the UK: Results of the Fourth National Audit Project of the Royal College of Anaesthetists and the Difficult Airway Society. Part 1: Anaesthesia. British Journal of Anaesthesia. 2011;**106**(5):617-631

[21] Adewale L. Anatomy and assessment of the pediatric airway. Paediatric Anaesthesia. 2009;**19**(Suppl 1):1-8

[22] Jenkins IA, Saunders M. Infections of the airway. Paediatric Anaesthesia. 2009;**19**(Suppl 1): 118-130

[23] Infosino A. Pediatric upper airway and congenital anomalies. Anesthesiology Clinics of North America. 2002;**20**(4):747-766

[24] Practice guidelines for management of the difficult airway. A report by the American Society of Anesthesiologists Task Force on Management of the Difficult Airway. Anesthesiology. 1993;**78**(3):597-602

[25] Samsoon GL, Young JR. Difficult tracheal intubation: A retrospective study. Anaesthesia. 1987;**42**(5):487-490

[26] Santos AP, Mathias LA, Gozzani JL, Watanabe M. Difficult intubation in children: Applicability of the Mallampati index. Revista Brasileira de Anestesiologia. 2011;**61**(2): 156-158 159-162, 184-187

[27] Miller DM. A proposed classification and scoring system for supraglottic sealing airways: A brief review. Anesthesia & Analgesia. 2004;**99**(5):1553-1559; Table of contents

[28] Brain AI, Verghese C, Strube PJ. The LMA 'ProSeal'–A laryngeal mask with an oesophageal vent. British Journal of Anaesthesia. 2000;**84**(5):650-654

[29] Agro F, Frass M, Benumof JL, Krafft P. Current status of the combitube: A review of the literature. Journal of Clinical Anesthesia. 2002;**14**(4):307-314

[30] Practice guidelines for management of the difficult airway: An updated report by the American Society of Anesthesiologists Task Force on Management of the Difficult Airway. Anesthesiology. 2003;**98**(5):1269-1277

[31] Viswanathan S, Campbell C, Wood DG, Riopelle JM, Naraghi M. The eschmann tracheal tube introducer. (Gum elastic bougie). Anesthesiology Review. 1992;**19**(6):29-34

[32] Inoue Y. Lightwand intubation can improve airway management. Canadian Journal of Anaesthesia. 2004;**51**(10):1052-1053

[33] Imashuku Y, Kojima A, Takahashi K, Kitagawa H. Endotracheal intubation training for clinical trainees in Japan is the anesthesiology training not necessary? Journal of Clinical Anesthesia. 2016;**31**:34

[34] Madziala M, Okruznik M, Cobo SA, Almira EF, Smereka J. Gold rules for pediatric endotracheal intubation. American Journal of Emergency Medicine. 2016;**34**(8):1711-1712

[35] Sakurai Y, Tamura M. Efficacy of the Airway Scope (Pentax-AWS) for training in pediatric intubation. Pediatrics International. 2015;**57**(2):217-221

[36] Moussa A, Luangxay Y, Tremblay S, Lavoie J, Aube G, Savoie E, et al. Videolaryngoscope for teaching neonatal endotracheal intubation: A randomized controlled trial. Pediatrics. 2016;**137**(3):e20152156

[37] Johnston LC, Auerbach M, Kappus L, Emerson B, Zigmont J, Sudikoff SN. Utilization of exploration-based learning and video-assisted learning to teach GlideScope videolaryngoscopy. Teaching and Learning in Medicine. 2014;**26**(3):285-291

[38] Leung SK, Cruz AT, Macias CG, Sirbaugh PE, Patel B. Improving pediatric emergency care by implementing an eligible learner Endotracheal Intubation Policy. Pediatric Emergency Care. 2016;**32**(4):205-209

[39] Goto T, Gibo K, Hagiwara Y, Okubo M, Brown DF, Brown CA 3rd, et al. Factors Associated with first-pass success in pediatric intubation in the emergency department. The Western Journal of Emergency Medicine. 2016;**17**(2):129-134

[40] Dongara AR, Modi JJ, Nimbalkar SM, Desai RG. Proficiency of residents and fellows in performing neonatal intubation. Indian Pediatrics. 2014;**51**(7):561-564

[41] Downes KJ, Narendran V, Meinzen-Derr J, McClanahan S, Akinbi HT. The lost art of intubation: Assessing opportunities for residents to perform neonatal intubation. Journal of Perinatology. 2012;**32**(12):927-932

[42] Andreatta PB, Dooley-Hash SL, Klotz JJ, Hauptman JG, Biddinger B, House JB. Retention curves for pediatric and neonatal intubation skills after simulation-based training. Pediatric Emergency Care. 2016;**32**(2):71-76

[43] Andreatta PB, Klotz JJ, Dooley-Hash SL, Hauptman JG, Biddinger B, House JB. Performance-based comparison of neonatal intubation training outcomes: Simulator and live animal. Advances in Neonatal Care. 2015;**15**(1):56-64

http://dx.doi.org/10.5772/intechopen.70356

[44] Finan E, Bismilla Z, Campbell C, Leblanc V, Jefferies A, Whyte HE. Improved procedural performance following a simulation training session may not be transferable to the clinical environment. Journal of Perinatology. 2012;**32**(7):539-544

[45] Nishisaki A, Donoghue AJ, Colborn S, Watson C, Meyer A, Brown CA 3rd, et al. Effect of just-in-time simulation training on tracheal intubation procedure safety in the pediatric intensive care unit. Anesthesiology. 2010;**113**(1):214-223

Chapter 4

# Emergency Pericardiocentesis in Children

Cecilia Lazea

Additional information is available at the end of the chapter

http://dx.doi.org/10.5772/intechopen.70700

**Abstract**

Cardiac tamponade is a life-threatening condition characterized by compression of the heart due to pericardial accumulation of different types of fluid and requires prompt diagnosis and immediate therapeutic intervention. Echocardiography is the most useful imaging technique to diagnose the cardiac tamponade and to evaluate the size, location, and hemodynamic impact of the pericardial effusion. Emergency pericardiocentesis is the procedure used for the aspiration of the fluid from the pericardial space in patients with significant pericardial effusion which determines hemodynamic compromise (cardiac tamponade). Emergency pericardiocentesis in children is performed under local anesthesia and is echocardiographic-guided. The first step of echocardiographic-guided pericardiocentesis is to assess the dimension and distribution of the pericardial fluid and the optimal trajectory of the needle in order to efficiently evacuate the pericardial fluid. The transducer is situated 3–5 cm from the parasternal border and the trajectory of the needle is established by the angle of the transducer. The needle is positioned between the xiphoid process and the left costal cartilages and is advanced, while a continuous aspiration is performed. It is important to avoid the neighboring vital organs (heart, liver, lung, internal mammary artery, and the intercostal vascular bundle). Complications which can occur are as follows: dysrhythmias, puncture of coronary artery or mammary artery, hemothorax, pneumothorax, pneumopericardium, and hepatic injury.

**Keywords:** pericardiocentesis, emergency, children, cardiac tamponade

## 1. Introduction

Pericardiocentesis is indicated in hemodynamic unstable children with cardiac tamponade. Echocardiography is a useful imaging tool for liquid effusion visualization and for needle trajectory, reducing the risk of complications.

## 2. Cardiac tamponade

### 2.1. Definition

Cardiac tamponade is a life-threatening condition characterized by compression of the heart due to pericardial accumulation of different types of fluid in the pericardial space, which determines restriction from normal filling of the cardiac chambers. Other causes that can determine cardiac tamponade are as follows: inflammation, trauma, aortic dissection, and rupture of the heart [1]. This condition requires prompt diagnosis and immediate therapeutic intervention.

### 2.2. Etiology

Cardiac tamponade can appear in children as a result of the following conditions (**Table 1**).

Accumulation of transudative fluid into pericardial space can occur from obstruction of fluid drainage, while exudative fluid accumulation appears secondary to inflammation, infections, autoimmune, and malignant diseases.

### 2.3. Physiopathology

Pericardium envelops the heart and consists of two layers (the visceral pericardium and the parietal pericardium), which are separated by a virtual space containing a small amount of fluid (about 20 mL), serving as lubricant. Normally, pericardium has little effect on cardiovascular function as the following: preservation of the interaction between the left and right ventricle during the systole and diastole, limitation of the intrathoracic cardiac movement and acute cardiac dilatation, minimization of the friction between the heart and neighboring structures by the presence of a small amount of fluid in the pericardial space, and anatomic barrier for pulmonary infections by lymphatic structure [1–3].

Abnormal pericardial fluid production will determine an increased intrapericardial pressure, when the normal capacitance volume of the pericardium is exceeded, with hemodynamic

| Common causes | Uncommon causes |
|---|---|
| Infectious pericardial effusion (viral, pyogenic, tuberculous) | Postcardiac percutaneous procedures |
| Uremia | Radiofrequency ablation |
| Neoplasia (metastases, leukemia, lymphoma) | Transvenous pacemaker lead implantation |
| Postcardiac surgery (postpericardiotomy syndrome) | Radiation therapy |
| Collagen vascular diseases (systemic lupus erythematosus) | Chemotherapy |
| Trauma (hemopericardum) | Myocardial infarction |
| | Aortic dissection |
| | Hypothyroidism |
| | Kawasaki disease |
| | Juvenile idiopathic arthritis |
| | Rheumatic fever |

**Table 1.** Causes of cardiac tamponade [1–8].

consequences, depending on the rate of liquid accumulation in the pericardial sac. Slow accumulation of the fluid cannot produce clinical symptoms, even when a large quantity of fluid is present, while a rapid accumulation of pericardial fluid will determine a sudden increase of the intrapericardial pressure with severe clinical and hemodynamic consequences. Cardiac tamponade can appear in case of sudden increase of the intrapericardial fluid volume or in case of progressive increase of the pericardial fluid beyond the point of possible pericardial distension. In cardiac tamponade, the diastolic filling is severely reduced because of the increased intrapericardial pressure and conversely, the cardiac output will be reduced. During inspiration, the right ventricle is expanded because of the increased inflow, while during expiration, the left ventricle is expanded and causes the diastolic collapse of the right ventricle and right atrium [2, 3, 9, 10].

### 2.4. Clinical presentation

During the initial stages, ejection fraction and heart rate are increased and consecutively, the cardiac output is preserved. Lately, the compensatory mechanisms are not effective and systemic vascular resistance are increased, in order to maintain systemic blood pressure, with systemic perfusion compromising and finally with decreased myocardial function, reduced cardiac output, and blood pressure. Clinically, the Beck's triad expresses these pathophysiological changes described above and consists of distant heart sounds, hypotension, and jugular venous distension because of elevated central venous pressure. Other clinical signs are diminished peripheral pulses, pulsus paradoxus (a decrease in systolic blood pressure of >10 mmHg during inspiration), hepatomegaly, and Kussmaul's sign (increased jugular venous pressure during inspiration). In late phases, cyanosis and decreased level of consciousness can be present [1–3, 9–11].

### 2.5. Diagnosis

Cardiac tamponade is diagnosed clinically and on echocardiography, but there are other useful diagnostic investigations.

#### *2.5.1. Chest radiography*

Chest radiography can reveal an increased cardiac silhouette ("water-bottle" shape) or a normal-appearing cardiac silhouette.

#### *2.5.2. Electrocardiography*

Decreased electrocardiographic voltage and electric alternans (alternating P wave, QRS complex, and T wave voltages because of the swinging motion of the heart) are characteristics of cardiac tamponade.

#### *2.5.3. Echocardiography*

Echocardiography is the most useful imaging technique to diagnose the cardiac tamponade and to evaluate the size, location, and hemodynamic impact of the pericardial effusion. Emergency echocardiographic assessment of tamponade includes two stages: first stage demonstrates the presence of pericardial fluid collection and the second stage assesses the hemodynamic effects of previously detected collection [12]. The first sign of hemodynamic impairment in tamponade is collapse of the right ventricle free wall in early- to mid-diastole because of the increased intrapericardial pressure more than ventricular transmural distending pressure, and is very specific (**Figure 1**). Right atrial collapse appears in late diastole and has high specificity. The absence of the right chamber collapse is present in cases of elevated diastolic pressure in the right chambers, such as pulmonary hypertension, positive pressure ventilation, or severe left ventricle failure [9]. When tamponade progresses, left atrial late-diastolic collapse and left ventricle early-diastolic collapse can appear. Dilatation of inferior vena cava without normal inspiratory variation (less than 50% decrease in diameter during inspiration), known as inferior vena cava plethora, has also high sensitivity for cardiac tamponade. Other signs are swinging heart, respiratory variation in ventricular chamber size, pseudosystolic anterior motion of the mitral valve, fluttering of the ventricular septum, and dilated hepatic veins [1–4, 10, 12–15]. The absence of the heart chamber collapse is considered as a negative predictive sign for cardiac tamponade [9].

Cardiac tamponade occurring after open-heart surgery is suspected in case of signs of low cardiac output, fall in systemic blood pressure associated with tachycardia and increased

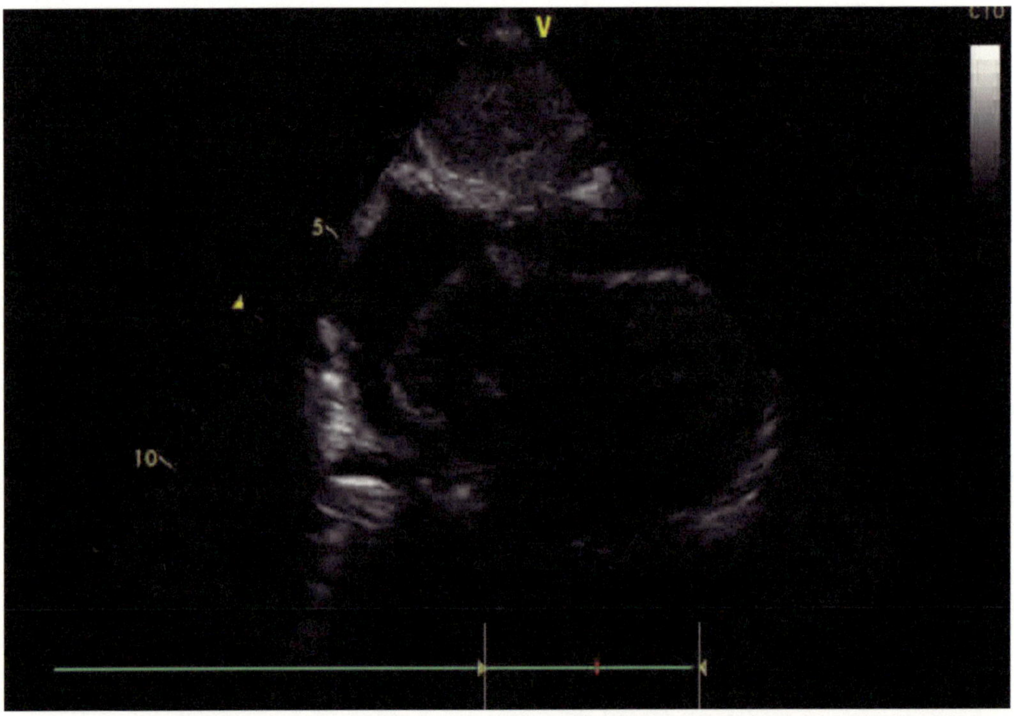


**Figure 1.** Tamponade, collapse of the right ventricle free wall (echocardiography—subcostal view).

filling pressure, oliguria, decrease of chest drainage, pulsus paradoxus, cardiac arrest, and widen mediastinal shadow on chest radiography [16].

Doppler echocardiography is another useful tool for diagnosis of tamponade, showing large variations with respiration (more than 30%) in the amplitude of inflow and outflow signals, as follows [1–3, 9, 10, 12–15].

- Mitral valve: exaggerated decrease in mitral inflow (E wave velocity) during inspiration and relatively increase of the atrial component (A wave velocity).
- Tricuspid valve: exaggerated increase in tricuspid inflow (E wave velocity) during inspiration.
- Peak velocities in left and right outflow tracts have a large difference with respiratory cycle. During inspiration, there is a drop of peak velocity in the aorta, while in the right ventricular outflow tract, there is an increase of peak velocity.
- Pulmonary veins: decrease of D wave velocity during inspiration.
- Hepatic veins: increased S wave velocity during inspiration; decreased or absence of D wave and high reversal during expiration.

Although there are many echocardiographic signs, none of these findings are entirely diagnostic of cardiac tamponade, so the diagnosis is based on both clinical and ultrasound assessment.

#### *2.5.4. Cardiac CT*

Cardiac CT can identify the collapse of the cardiac chambers.

#### *2.5.5. Cardiac MRI*

Cardiac MRI can identify the hemodynamic changes of tamponade (collapse of the cardiac chambers).

### 2.6. Treatment

Emergency pericardiocentesis represents the method used to relieve tamponade. Improvement of the blood pressure and cardiac output can be the result of removal even a small amount of fluid (except of the cases of purulent or malignant pericardial effusions).

## 3. Pericardiocentesis

### 3.1. Definition

Emergency pericardiocentesis is the procedure used for the aspiration of the fluid from the pericardial space in patients with significant pericardial effusion, which determines hemodynamic compromise (cardiac tamponade).

Pericardiotomy was first performed in 1815, and the subxiphoid approach was first described in 1911. The ultrasound-guided pericardiocentesis is considered the standard procedure because of lower rate of complications.

### 3.2. Indications

Pericardiocentesis is indicated in hemodynamic-unstable children with cardiac tamponade and to diagnose the cause of the presence of a pericardial fluid accumulation.

### 3.3. Contraindications

There are relative contraindications such as uncorrected bleeding disorders, anticoagulation therapy, thrombocytopenia, small pericardial effusion with posterior localization, and aortic dissection.

### 3.4. Equipment for pericardiocentesis

- Ultrasound machine (**Figure 2**)
- Cardiac monitor
- ECG machine
- Resuscitation equipment including defibrillator
- Antiseptic substances
- Local anesthetic
- Needles
- Syringes
- Catheter guide
- Seldinger wire
- Pigtail catheter
- Alligator clamps
- Drain tubes
- Collection system
- Sterile compressor for transducer
- Sterile fields
- Compresses

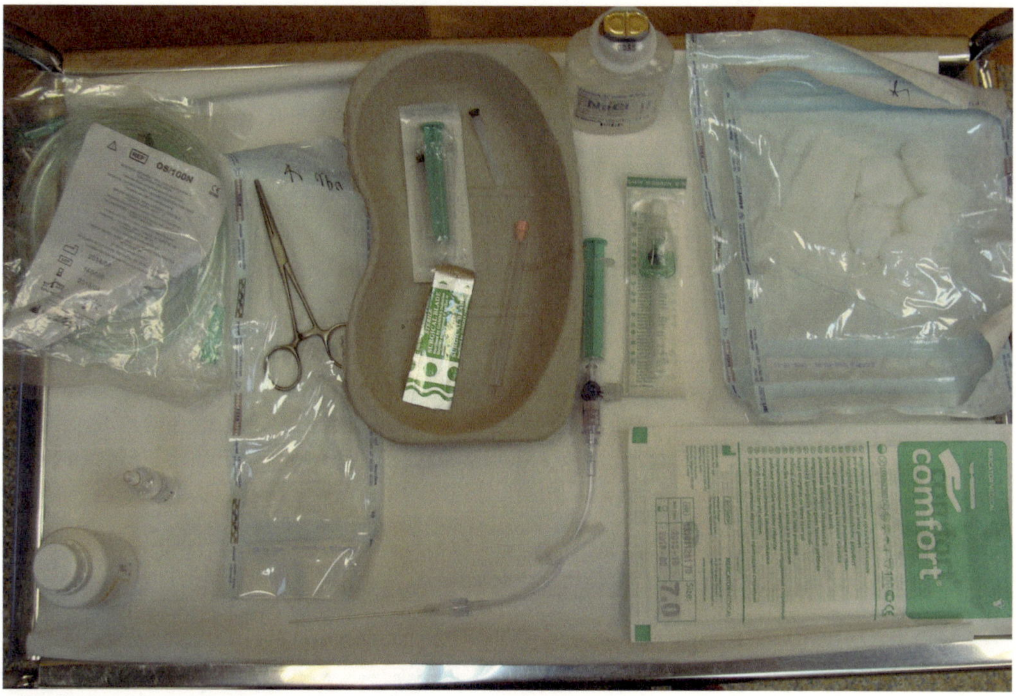


**Figure 2.** Equipment for pericardiocentesis.

### 3.5. Technique

*3.5.1. Preparation*

All equipment must be prepared before starting the procedure and full resuscitation equipment including defibrillator must be available. The patient must be attached to a cardiac monitor and must have an IV line in place. Sedation is necessary in patients who are awake. In patients who are unresponsive, sedation can produce hemodynamic or respiratory deterioration. It is also necessary to assure the availability for operating room in case of anatomic approach failure or consecutive complications.

Position at 45° can bring the heart closer to the thoracic anterior wall and is preferred in patients with stable clinical conditions. In case of distended abdomen, a nasogastric tube should be put in place. The platelet count and coagulation profile should be checked before the procedure [17, 18].

Sterile skin preparation and area disinfection are effectuated using betadine or other antiseptic substance, and sterile fields are used to isolate this area. Local anesthesia is recommended to be done by infiltration with 1% lidocaine.

*3.5.2. Anatomic approach*

Three main approaches such as the subxiphoid approach, parasternal approach, and apical approach are used, which are selected based on imaging guidance to find the maximum layer of effusion and avoiding the puncture of other structures [2, 10, 17–19].

***Subxiphoid (subcostal) approach*** was preferred for a long period of time and is the safest approach in cases without ultrasound guidance. The needle is inserted between the xiphoid process and the left costal margin at an angle of 30–45° to the skin, and is directed toward the left shoulder (**Figures 3** and **4**).

***Parasternal approach***: the needle is placed perpendicular to the skin in the fifth intercostal parasternal space, at 1–3 cm to the sternal border (to avoid the puncture of internal mammary artery). The needle is placed into the intercostal space above the superior edge of the rib (in order to avoid the neurovascular bundle, which is located inferiorly). The risk for pneumothorax is higher than using other approaches.

***Apical approach***: the needle is introduced 1 cm lateral to the apex beat or at the edge of cardiac dullness and is directed toward the right shoulder.

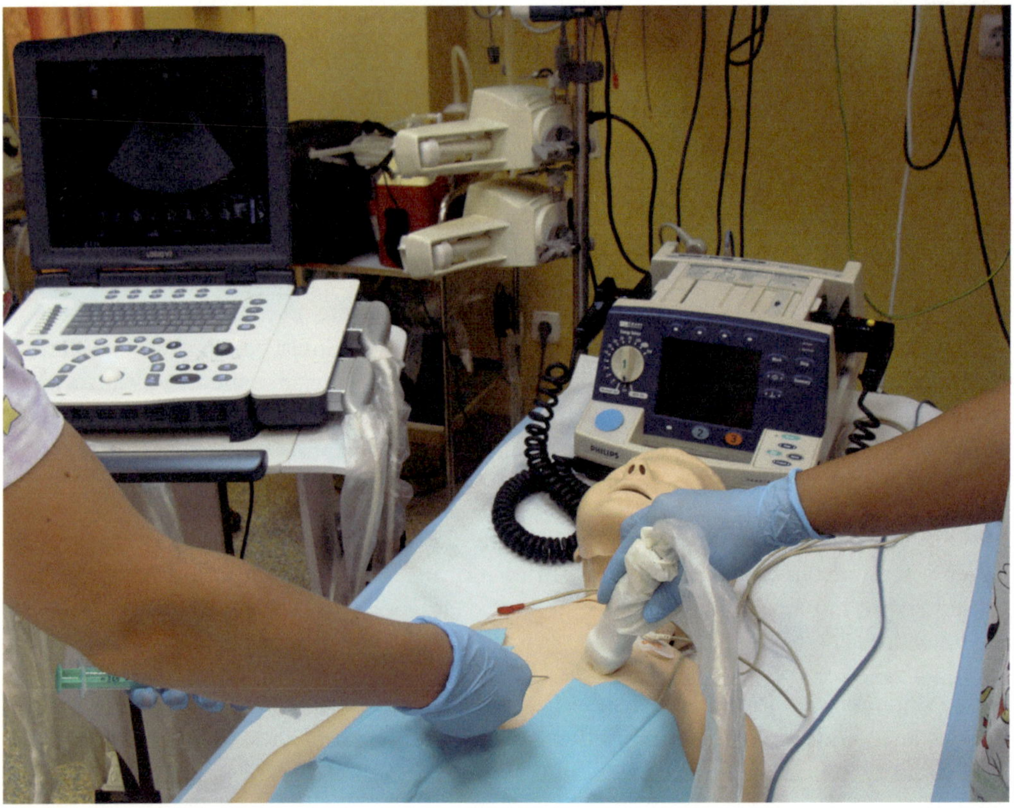


**Figure 3.** Echocardiographic-guided pericardiocentesis using the subxiphoid approach.

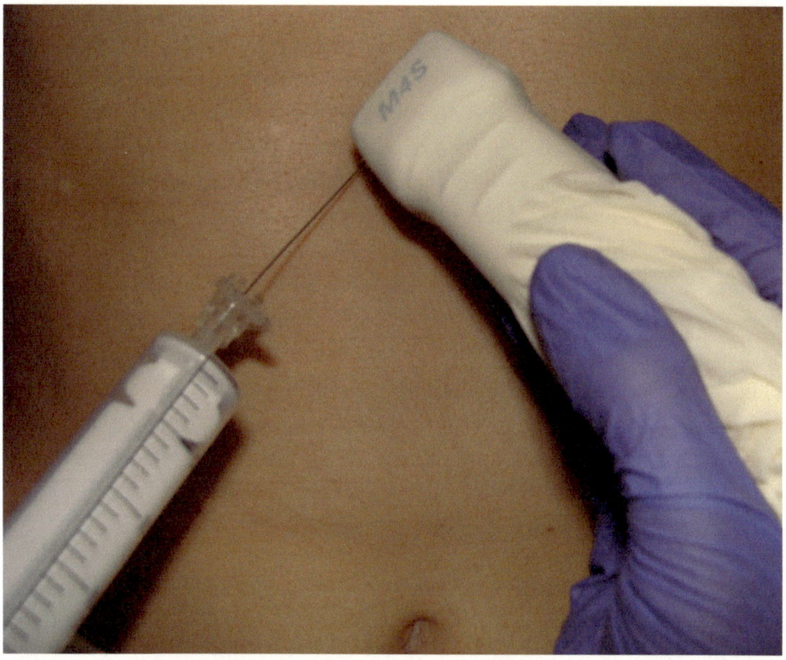


**Figure 4.** Echocardiographic-guided pericardiocentesis: needle insertion.

In both subxiphoid and sternal approaches, preferable patient's position is sitting at 45° angle, if the clinical condition permits, while supine position is used in patients with severe clinical condition [17, 20].

The advantages and disadvantages of these approaches are presented in **Table 2** [17, 21].

| Approach | Advantages | Disadvantages |
|---|---|---|
| Subxiphoid | The safest approach in unguided-pericardiocentesis<br>Low risk of pleural injury | High risk for hepatic, gastric, phrenic, and diaphragmatic damage |
| Parasternal | Echocardiography provides good visualization of the zone of maximum pericardial collection | High risk for pneumothorax and internal thoracic vessels injury |
| Apical | Lower risk of bleeding because of the paucity of cardiac vascularization near the heart apex<br>Left ventricle has thick walls and protects against puncture<br>No pleura near the apex and low risk of pneumothorax | Avoid in emergency situations |

**Table 2.** Pericardiocentesis approaches.

### *3.5.3. Procedure*

Emergency pericardiocentesis in children is recommended to be performed under echocardiographic guide. Blind pericardiocentesis is performed only in very rare situations, which are immediate life-threatening, because of the major risk for severe complications.

*3.5.3.1. Echocardiographic-guided pericardiocentesis*

The first step of echocardiographic-guided pericardiocentesis is to assess the dimension and distribution of the pericardial fluid and the optimal trajectory of the needle in order to efficiently evacuate the pericardial fluid. The area of maximal fluid accumulation is also determined using the echocardiography. The echocardiographic transducer is covered with a sterile material (sterile glove with ultrasound sterile gel) and is positioned approximately 3–5 cm from the left parasternal border, and the area of maximal fluid accumulation is identified. The direction and trajectory of needle follows the angle of the transducer. The place of puncture is delimitated by the angle between the xiphoid process and the left costal cartilages, and 18 mm gauge needles are recommended. The distance between the skin and pericardium is about 5 cm in children. The needle is directed at a 15° posterior angle toward the shoulder and is advanced, while a continuous aspiration is performed with a syringe and the fluid is obtained. The drainage is also assessed using the echocardiography [2, 10, 17–19].

*3.5.3.2. Pericardiocentesis with electrocardiographic assistance*

This procedure can be used when echocardiography guiding is not available. Electrocardiogram monitoring is begun after the pericardial space has been reached, before the needle is advanced. A sterile electrical cord is attached to the needle using an alligator clips and is connected to any precordial lead in order to avoid the ventricular puncture. The electrocardiographic mark of epicardium touching is a wide complex (like a premature ventricular complex, with elevated ST segment), known as current of injury pattern. Atrial arrhythmia or PR segment elevation shows the contact with atrial pericardium, while ventricular arrhythmia is the marker of mechanical stimulation of the ventricular epicardium. The current of injury appears when the needle touches the epicardium and from this point, there is a high risk of myocardium or coronary laceration. Until the current of injury disappears, the needle must be withdrawn few millimeters and then safely placed into the pericardial space [17].

*3.5.3.3. Fluid aspiration*

Aspiration of pericardial fluid can increase the risk of cardiac puncture. Nonclotting aspirated blood and a lower hematocrit level may indicate a pericardial origin [17]. Diagnostic studies are performed on pericardial fluid such as cell count, protein level, glucose, lactate dehydrogenase, bacterial, fungal, and mycobacterial culture, viral PCR, and tumor cytology.

*3.5.3.4. Percutaneous pericardial drainage*

Insertion of a drainage catheter is used to avoid and to reduce the rate of recurrence. The subxiphoid approach is recommended using an 18-mm gauge needle. After the pericardial puncture, the position of the needle in the pericardial sac is assessed using 5–6 mL of agitated saline solution, which is injected and monitored by echocardiography, confirming the position of needle (microbubbles will create contrast into pericardial fluid). A guide wire is inserted into the pericardial space and the needle is removed, and dilatation of the needle tract is performed. Then, a pigtail catheter is inserted over the guide wire via the Seldinger technique and is left in place for few days for drainage of chronic effusions [2, 10, 13, 17, 19].

### 3.6. Complications

Complications which can occur are as follows: dysrhythmias (atrial fibrillation, ventricular tachycardia, asystole), puncture of coronary artery, hemothorax, pneumothorax, pneumopericardium, cardiac laceration, epicardial or pericardial thrombus, ventricular dysfunction, arterial hypotension because of vasovagal reaction, sudden pulmonary edema due to a sudden increase in pulmonary return, circulatory collapse in patients with an increased rate of drainage, lung laceration, intercostal vessels injury, mammary artery injury, pleuropericardic fistula, infection, diaphragm, phrenic, gastric and hepatic injury, and hemoperitoneum [2, 10, 17–21].

### 3.7. Follow-up

After pericardiocentesis, an individualized follow-up is required. Daily echocardiographic evaluation is performed in the first few days during hospitalization to evaluate pericardial effusion recurrence and weekly evaluation after patient discharge is required [13].

***Tips and tricks:***

- Diagnostic of cardiac tamponade is based on both clinical and ultrasound assessment.
- When the needle penetrates the pericardium, the patient who is awake can undergo a sharp chest pain.
- During pericardiocentesis, the needle should not be further advanced after aspiration of pericardial fluid.
- If a large quantity of blood is aspirated, the needle could be in the ventricle.
- Clotting fluid does not reliably indicate the position of needle.
- An increased rate of drainage can determine circulatory collape.

## Author details

Cecilia Lazea

Address all correspondence to: cicilazearo@yahoo.com

Department of Pediatrics I, "Iuliu Hatieganu" University of Medicine and Pharmacy, Cluj-Napoca, Romania

## References

[1] Adler Y, Charron P, Imazio M, Badano L, Barón-Esquivias G, Bogaert J, Brucato A, Gueret P, Klingel K, Lionis C, Maisch B, Mayosi B, Pavie A, Ristić AD, Sabaté Tenas M, Seferovic P, Swedberg K, Tomkowski W, Achenbach S, Agewall S, Al-Attar N, Angel Ferrer J, Arad M, Asteggiano R, Bueno H, Caforio AL, Carerj S, Ceconi C, Evangelista A, Flachskampf F,

Giannakoulas G, Gielen S, Habib G, Kolh P, Lambrinou E, Lancellotti P, Lazaros G, Linhart A, Meurin P, Nieman K, Piepoli MF, Price S, Roos-Hesselink J, Roubille F, Ruschitzka F, Sagristà Sauleda J, Sousa-Uva M, Uwe Voigt J, Luis Zamorano J. 2015 ESC Guidelines for the diagnosis and management of pericardial diseases. European Heart Journal. 2015;**36**(42):2921-2964. DOI: 10.1093/eurheartj/ehv318

[2] Tissot C, Phelps C, da Cruz E, Miyamoto S. Pericardial diseases. In: Munoz R, Morrel V, da Cruz E, Vetterly C, editors. Critical Care of Children with Heart Disease. 1st ed. London: Springer-Verlag; 2010. p. 521-541. DOI: 10.1007/978-1-84882-262-7

[3] Johnson J, Cetta F. Pericardial diseases. In: Allen H, Driscoll D, Shaddy R, Feltes T, editors. Moss and Adams' Heart Disease in Infants, Children, and Adolescents Including the Fetus and Young Adult. 8th ed. Philadelphia: Lippincott Williams & Wilkins, Wolters Kluwer; 2013. p. 1350-1362

[4] American Heart Association. Pediatric Advanced Life Support. USA: First American Heart Association Printing; 2016. p. 352

[5] Arabi MT, Malek EM, Fares MH, Itani MH. Cardiac tamponade as the first manifestation of lupus erithematosus in children. BMJ Case Reports. 2012; DOI: 10.1136/bcr-2012-006927

[6] Simbre VC, Duffy SA, Dadlani GH, Miller TL, Lipshultz SE. Cardiotoxicity of cancer chemotherapy: Implications for children. Paediatric Drugs. 2005;**7**(3):187-202

[7] Goldenberg J, Pessoa AP, Roizenblatt S, Pavoa RM, Hilario MO, Atra E, Ferraz MB. Cardiac tamponade in juvenile chronic arthritis: Report of two cases and review of publications. Annals of the Rheumatic Diseases. 1990;**49**(7):549-553

[8] Akikusa JD. Rheumatologic emergencies in newborns, children, and adolescents. Pediatric Clinics of North America. 2012;**59**(2):285-299. DOI: 10.1016/j.pcl.2012.03.001

[9] Perez-Casares A, Cesar S, Brunet-Garcia L, Sanchez-de-Toledo J. Echocardiographic evaluation of pericardial effusion and cardiac tamponade. Frontiers in Pediatrics. 2017. DOI: 10.3389/fped.2017.00079

[10] Tissot C. Pericardial Diseases. In: Da Cruz E, Ivy D, Jaggers J, editors. Pediatric and Congenital Cardiology, Cardiac Surgery and Intensive Care. 1st ed. London: Springer-Verlag; 2014. p. 2369-2394. DOI: 10.1007/978-1-4471-4619-3

[11] Johnson W, Moller J. Pediatric Cardiology. The Essential Pocket Guide. 3rd ed. Oxford: Wiley Blackwell; 2014. 392 p

[12] Tavazzi G, Price S. Ecocardiography in the intensive care unit. In: Berstein A, Soni N, editors. OH's Intensive Care Manual. 7th ed. China: Elsevier; 2014. p. 308-323

[13] Cosyns B, Plein S, Nihoyanopoulos P, Smiseth O, Achenbach S, Andrade MJ, Pepi M, Ristic A, Imazio M, Paelinck B, Lancellotti P, European Association of Cardiovascular Imaging (EACVI); European Society of Cardiology Working Group (ESC WG) on Myocardial and Pericardial diseases. European Association of Cardiovascular Imaging

(EACVI) position paper: Multimodality imaging in pericardial disease. European Heart Journal. Cardiovascular Imaging. 2015;**16**(1):12-31. DOI: 10.1093/ehjci/jeu128

[14] Leeson P, Becher H. Pericardial effusion and cardiac tamponade. In: Zamorano JL, Bax J, Knuuti J, Sechtem U, Lancellotti P, Badano L, editors. The ESC Textbook of Cardiovascular Imaging. 2nd ed. New York: Oxford University Press; 2015. p. 509-519

[15] Gaspar HA, Morhy S. The role of focused echocardiography in pediatric intensive care: A critical appraisal. BioMed Research International. 2015. DOI: 10.1155/2015/596451

[16] Shah P. Manual of Pediatric Cardiac Intensive Care. 1st ed. New Delhi: Jaypee Brothers Medical Publishers Ltd; 2013. 159 p

[17] Harper R. Pericardiocentesis. In: Roberts J, Hedges J, editors. Clinical Procedures in Emergency Medicine. 4th ed. Philadelphia: Saunders; 2004. p. 305-322

[18] Synovitz C, Brown E. Pericardiocentesis. In: Tintinalli J, Stapczynski S, Ma J, Yealy D, Meckler G, Cline D, editors. Tintinalli's Emergency Medicine: A Comprehensive Study Guide. 8th ed. USA: McGraw-Hill; 2016. p. 236-242

[19] Gewitz M, Satou G, Wheeler D. Diseases of the pericardium. In: Wheeler D, Wong H, Shanley T, editors. Pediatric Critical Care Medicine. Basic Science and Clinical Evidence. 1st ed. London: Springer-Verlag; 2007. p. 821-828

[20] Gluer R, Murdoch D, Haqqani M, Scalia G, Walters D. Pericardiocentesis—How to do it. Heart, Lung & Circulation. 2015;**24**(6):621-625. DOI: 10. 1016/j.hlc.2014.11.009

[21] Kumar R. Complications of pericardiocentesis: A clinical synopsis. International Journal of Critical Illness and Injury Science. 2015;**5**(3):206-212. DOI: 10.4103/2229-5151.165007

Chapter 5

# Lumbar Puncture of the Newborn

Selim Öncel

Additional information is available at the end of the chapter

http://dx.doi.org/10.5772/intechopen.70498

**Abstract**

Heinrich Irenäus Quincke was the first person in medical history to perform lumbar puncture (LP). Indications of lumbar puncture include suspected meningitis, suspected subarachnoid hemorrhage, administration of chemotherapeutic agents, instillation of contrast media for imaging of the spinal cord, and the evaluation of various neurologic conditions including normal pressure hydrocephalus and Guillain-Barré syndrome, and the treatment of idiopathic intracranial hypertension. Contraindications of lumbar puncture include findings of increased intracranial pressure, bleeding diathesis, cardiopulmonary instability, soft tissue infection at the puncture site, shock, respiratory insufficiency, and suspected meningococcal septicemia with extensive or spreading purpura. Altered mental status, focal neurologic signs, papilledema, focal seizure, and risk for brain abscess are indications for cranial imaging before performing LP. Lack of local anesthetic use and advancement of the spinal needle with the stylet in place were most prominent risk factors for a traumatic LP. Ultrasound may minimize the number of LP attempts and decrease patient and parent anxiety by easily identifying an insertion site. Infection, spinal hematoma, epidermoid tumor, and cerebral herniation are the main complications of LP. When LP is traumatic, the wisest approach is to assume the patient is having meningitis and start empirical therapy.

**Keywords:** infants, neonate, newborns, lumbar puncture, spinal tap, meningitis

## Core tips

It seems that Heinrich Irenäus Quincke was the first person in medical history to use lumbar puncture for therapeutic, and subsequently, diagnostic purposes.

Empirical antibiotic therapy for suspected meningitis, which should ideally succeed lumbar puncture, should be started immediately if lumbar puncture is to be delayed.

Lumbar puncture should always be performed as soon as the infant becomes clinically stable and can tolerate the procedure even if it has not been possible to be performed at the first suspicion of meningitis.

Lumbar puncture can be performed safely in patients with thrombocytopenia less than 10,000/μL, if they receive transfusion to a peripheral platelet count greater than 50,000/μL, and in patients with coagulopathy after appropriate correction of factor deficiency.

Physicians may have to treat suspected meningitis being deprived of cerebrospinal fluid (CSF) analysis guidance, since getting parental consent for lumbar puncture may be problematic.

During lumbar puncture, airway and resuscitation equipment should be immediately at hand.

Lumbar puncture in children younger than 12 months must be performed below the L2-L3 interspace.

The presence of a family member was found to be associated with neither an increased risk of traumatic or unobtainable lumbar puncture nor more attempts at the procedure.

The "ideal" angle for lumbar puncture as determined with ultrasonography was 50° in infants in both the lateral recumbent and sitting positions.

When lumbar puncture is traumatic, the wisest approach is to assume the patient as having meningitis and start empirical therapy.

## 1. Introduction

Lumbar puncture (LP) may be considered one of the most well-known diagnostic procedures in the field of pediatric infectious diseases. It is an essential procedure for analyzing cerebrospinal fluid (CSF) in the evaluation for meningitis, sepsis, fever, or subarachnoid hemorrhage (SAH) in neonates.

## 2. History

Our knowledge of meninges dates back to ancient Egypt, where it was described in Ebers papyrus around 1500 BC. Hippocrates (and his physician contemporaries) must have been aware of the presence of CSF, since he is known to have referred to hydrocephalus as "water in the head."

Despite, apparently, a long time has passed since the discovery of CSF, its usual collection technique, called lumbar puncture, has a relatively short history—about only a century long. The answer to the question of who has performed the first lumbar puncture is still a little matter of debate today:

- In 1885, North-American neurologist Leonard Corning (1855–1923) published two articles, in which he described the application of "local medication" cocaine for local anesthesia to the spinal cord in thoracic D1–D2 interspace, most probably in the epidural space not removing any CSF.

- Heinrich Irenäus Quincke (1842–1922), a German professor of internal medicine in Kiel, presented his first communication on LP in the "X. Kongress der Gesellschaft für inneren Medizin" (X. Congress of the Society of Internal Medicine) in Wiesbaden, Germany on April 8, 1891. In his first procedure of its kind, Quincke used a hollow needle with stiletto, which very closely resembles the LP needles that are routinely used today. He entered the subarachnoid space at the L3-L4 intervertebral level and drained CSF with the purpose of relieving headache, suffered by children with hydrocephalus. Quincke coined the term "Lumbalpunction" (LP) in his subsequent paper on this field.
- According to English physician Walter Essex Wynter's (1860–1945) article published in the Lancet on May 2, 1891, he made a skin incision at the second lumbar vertebra, and then made a big opening up to the dura mater, in addition to which laminectomy was often required. Next, he introduced a trochar and took CSF out for decreasing CSF pressure. Wynter used the term "paracentesis" for his procedure.

It is clearly seen that all three investigators have done the procedure for therapeutic, not diagnostic purposes, which is the main difference from today's LP. It is also obvious that Corning's performance involves a site (thoracic) and an intermeningeal space (epidural) that is very distinct from LP.

Although some authors mention the names of Corning and Wynter, it seems that Quincke was the first person in medical history to use LP for therapeutic, and subsequently, diagnostic purposes. Putting the common point of therapeutic use apart, during the time of publication, characteristics of puncture and nomenclature used were compared; we, in agreement with authors like Frederiks and Koehler, favor Quincke as the discoverer of LP. Besides, we believe that he deserves this title for being the first investigator to apply LP for diagnostic purposes thereafter [1, 2].

## 3. Indications

- The main indication for LP in newborn period is suspected central nervous system (CNS) infection. LP is an indispensable and emergent tool in the diagnosis of neonatal meningitis and should ideally precede the initiation of empirical antimicrobial therapy. If LP should be delayed or cannot be performed for any reason, such as deteriorating clinical status of the patient or transferring the patient to another health institution, empirical antibiotic therapy should be started immediately, since minutes count in the diagnosis and early commencement of therapy [3].

Clinical findings of neonatal meningitis are similar to those of neonatal sepsis with or without meningitis. Thus, it is not possible to predict with physical findings alone whether the infant has sepsis, meningitis, or both. Although signs of sepsis and meningitis intertwine in the newborn period, some neonatologist deem it unnecessary to perform LP on neonates evaluated for sepsis, especially those with early neonatal sepsis [4, 5], because the antibiotics for both conditions would be the same. However, it should be kept in mind that blood cultures are negative in one-third of neonates with meningitis who are very-low-birth-weight and born over 34 weeks of gestation [6]. Thus, in case of LP is not performed, a significant portion of neonates with meningitis would not get a correct diagnosis and would not be observed for the likely complications of meningitis. For that reason, the author is in favor of the opinion that LP should always be performed as soon as the infant becomes clinically stable and can tolerate the procedure even if it has not been possible to be performed at the first suspicion of meningitis. CSF inflammation lasts for a considerably long duration of days, which would allow the clinician to diagnose or exclude the diagnosis of meningitis although CSF cultures may become negative within hours.

- Suspected subarachnoid hemorrhage (SAH) is another emergent indication for LP. Computed tomography (CT) should be performed for all children suspected of having SAH. There are times when SAH is not detectable on a CT scan and LP becomes the sole method of diagnosing this condition [7].
- Other indications for LP include the administration of chemotherapeutic agents, instillation of contrast media for imaging of the spinal cord, and the evaluation of various neurologic conditions including normal pressure hydrocephalus and Guillain-Barré syndrome. Among therapeutic uses of LP, removal of CSF in the treatment of idiopathic intracranial hypertension (pseudotumor cerebri) is noteworthy [8].

## 4. Contraindications

A contraindication to LP can be absolute or relative. In all situations, the clinician should use her/his clinical judgment by taking into account the relative risk of performing LP.

- Increased intracranial pressure (ICP): Increased intracranial pressure (ICP) is an absolute contraindication. Children with elevated ICP are at risk for cerebral herniation during LP. Therefore, cranial CT of all patients with clinical suspicion of increased ICP is essential for the physician's decision to perform LP, including those at risk because of brain abscess [8].
- Bleeding diathesis: Our knowledge regarding the safety of performing LP in patients with thrombocytopenia or coagulation factor deficiency is limited. The safety of LP in thrombocytopenia was investigated in 5223 LPs performed on 958 children with acute lymphoblastic leukemia in a retrospective study. Of these LPs, 912 were done at platelet counts of 11,000–20,000/μL, and 29 were performed at platelet counts of 10,000/μL or less. Serious complications of LP were not observed, regardless of platelet count. The authors concluded that prophylactic platelet transfusion was not necessary in children with platelet counts higher than 10,000/μL with a little caution that no conclusion can be made for children with platelet counts of 10,000/μL or less, due to the small number of patients in the study [9].

Because of the risk of subdural or epidural hematoma formation, many experts are against performing LP in patients with coagulation defects who are bleeding, severely thrombocytopenic (i.e., with platelet counts $<50,000/\mu L$), receiving anticoagulant therapy or an international normalized ratio of 1.4 or higher, without correcting the underlying abnormalities [8, 10]. However, LP can be performed safely in patients with thrombocytopenia less than 10,000/μL, if they receive transfusion to a peripheral platelet count greater than 50,000/μL, and in patients with coagulopathy after appropriate correction of factor deficiency [9, 11].

- Cardiopulmonary instability: The position of the newborn during LP may result in cardiopulmonary compromise. This issue will be addressed further in detail elsewhere in the text.
- Soft tissue infection at the puncture site
- Shock
- Respiratory insufficiency
- Suspected meningococcal septicemia with extensive or spreading purpura [10]

Conditions listed below are conditions in which imaging is needed before LP to exclude brain shift, swelling, or space occupying lesion [10]:

- Moderate to severe impairment of consciousness [Glascow coma scale (GCS) < 13 or 9 according to some experts] or fall in GCS of >2
- Focal neurological signs (including unequal, dilated, or poorly responsive pupils)
- Abnormal posture or posturing
- Papilledema
- After seizures until stabilized
- Relative bradycardia with hypertension
- Abnormal "doll's eye" movements
- Immunocompromise

Consequently, LP is sometimes contraindicated simply because the patient is too ill to safely undergo the procedure.

## 5. Parental consent

Since patients without appropriate decisional capacity cannot give their informed consent and written informed consent of the caregiver is required before the procedure, in many institutions including ours, it is customary for physicians to talk to parents for providing informed permission for an intervention like LP on their child. A straightforward explanation of the urgency and essentialness of the procedure, as well as the details of the procedure itself, maybe with the help of comparison with usual venipuncture (author's practice), is usually reassuring and should routinely be provided. Sometimes parents refuse to give assent and physicians are forced to initiate and continue CNS infection treatment totally blindfolded—that is without being able to include or exclude the diagnosis, grow the etiologic organism, and confirm the treatment success. Although LP is a relatively safe process, results from studies show that the most frequent concern that lay behind a dissent is that LP would cause a complication [12, 13]. In a single-center study carried out in Turkey, the most feared complication was paralysis (60%) followed by sterility (22%) [14].

## 6. Imaging

The decision to carry out imaging before LP should be done on a case-by-case basis. Children with the following conditions may have increased intracranial pressure (ICP) and, because of the assumption is that CT scan of the head can more or less reliably predict who will and who will not experience brain herniation after lumbar puncture, are advised to have a CT scan performed before LP [15]:

- Altered mental status
- Focal neurologic signs
- Papilledema
- Focal seizure
- Risk for brain abscess (immunocompromise or congenital heart disease with a right-to-left shunt)

It should be noted that a normal CT scan does not fully exclude the presence of elevated ICP or the possibility that elevated ICP will not develop thereafter. It is also known from adult studies that even those not undergoing LP because of a mass effect on head CTs may experience brain herniation [16]. Thus, although imaging for this purpose has been questioned by some specialists of this field, we agree with the recommendation that LP can be considered within 6 hours of a normal CT scan and no other contraindications [8, 17].

## 7. Preparation

Once the informed consent is obtained and imaging is performed if necessary, it is time for:

- providing oxygen saturation, respirations, and heart rate (HR) monitoring for critically-ill children during the procedure;
- "rehearsing" the position that infants will assume and getting help from a health care personnel who can hold the infant in sitting position if she/he is in respiratory distress (since in this position LP may be tolerated better) [18];
- getting help from a radiologist for patients with spinal abnormalities, such as spina bifida or severe scoliosis, to perform the procedure under ultrasonographic guidance [19]; and

- identification of infants who may require sedation or topical transdermal anesthesia for the procedure.

Materials needed for a smooth LP may be listed as follows [8]:

- Lidocaine 1% without epinephrine and topical anesthetic cream, such as liposomal lidocaine or eutectic mixture of lidocaine 2.5% and prilocaine 2.5%
- Sterile 3 mL syringe with 25-gauge needle for lidocaine injection
- Four sterile collecting tubes
- Sterile gloves
- Sterile drapes
- Povidone-iodine solution
- Sterile sponges for preparing puncture site
- Manometer (typically used in patients older than two years of age)
- 22-gauge and 1.5 inches (3.75 cm) long styletted spinal needle [7]
- Resuscitation equipment

## 8. Anatomy

CSF circulates in the space between the pia mater and the arachnoid mater, called subarachnoid space that surrounds the brain, spinal cord, ventricles, aqueductus cerebri (Sylvius), and central canal of the spinal cord. After the formation of most of its volume in the choroid plexuses of the lateral ventricles, CSF passes through the foramina of Luschka and Magendie into the subarachnoid space, which is around the spinal column and over the cerebrum. The CSF is primarily absorbed by the arachnoid villi found next to the sagittal sinus and then drains into the venous circulation [7, 20, 21]. In full-term infants, the volume of total CSF is about 40 mL, a quarter of which is in the ventricles, and the remainder in the subarachnoid space. CSF serves as a cushion between bony structures and the brain, together with the spinal cord. Since brain has no lymphatics, CSF also has an important role of carrying chemical byproducts of metabolism out of the brain to the venous circulation [7].

In order to avoid an accidental nervous injury, LP should be performed distal to the spinal cord, at the level of the cauda equina. In older children, LP can be performed from the L2-L3 interspace to the L5-S1 interspace, because these interspaces are below the termination of the spinal cord [8]. At birth, the inferior end of the spinal cord is opposite to the body of the third lumbar vertebra (L3); therefore, LP in children younger than 12 months must be performed below the L2-L3 interspace. As the child's spinal cord grows, the vertebral column grows more rapidly. An imaginary line that connects the two posterior-superior iliac crests intersects the spine at approximately the fourth lumbar vertebra. This landmark helps to locate the L3-L4 and L4-L5 interspaces [8]. Anatomic structures pierced during median LP in order are skin, subcutaneous fat, supraspinal ligament, interspinal ligament, ligamentum flavum, dura mater, and arachnoid mater [7].

## 9. Procedure

### 9.1. Before the procedure

Most of the time, LP is a relatively simple procedure, although it can sometimes prove challenging even for the most experienced physician. The potential for complications during and following LP makes it necessary that it be performed in an area with proper resuscitation equipment. Although not technically complex, LP is not a procedure that may be taken lightly, and it should only be performed by or under the supervision of a knowledgeable and experienced health professional.

HR, respiratory action, and oxygen saturation should be monitored closely during the procedure in neonates. Airway and resuscitation equipment should be immediately at hand. If the indication for the LP is elective, or by any other reason LP is not going to be done urgently, 4% lidocaine cream (effective after about 30 minutes) or eutectic mixture of lidocaine and prilocaine (effective after about 45–60 minutes) may be applied over the puncture site to lessen the pain [22, 23]. Due to the shorter time it takes for the onset of its effect, 4% lidocaine cream may be the preferred agent for this purpose.

### 9.2. Positioning of the newborn

According to a popular saying in pediatric circles in Turkey, "the person who performs the LP is the one who holds the infant." This saying emphasizes the challenging task of achieving and maintaining a proper patient position for the performer of LP. The patient is placed on the examining table. The goals of positioning are to stabilize the infant, to stretch the ligamenta flava and to increase the interlaminar spaces. The most common positions used for the pediatric LP are the lateral recumbent and sitting positions (**Figures 1** and **2**). For the lateral recumbent position, the patient is laid on her/his side near the edge of the bed. For a right-handed performer, the patient's head should face left because of ergonomics of the right upper extremity of the performer. The patient's neck is flexed and the knees are drawn up to the chest by the assistant by placing one arm under the child's knees and the other arm around the posterior aspect of the neck. The assistant should ensure that the spinal column is in no rotation by keeping the shoulders and hips perpendicular to the bed.

In the sitting position, the assistant holds the patient in the position with an arm and a leg in each hand while supporting the head to prevent from dropping, that is, excess flexion of the neck.

Choosing among the lateral recumbent and sitting positions with the neck or hip flexed or neutral, has not been standardized and is at the physician's disposal, and most neonatologists prefer placing the infant in lateral recumbent position [24]. The positions are important because they may be superior over one another in avoiding a traumatic tap (peripheral blood staining the CSF specimen) and to get sufficient amount of cerebrospinal fluid, which should

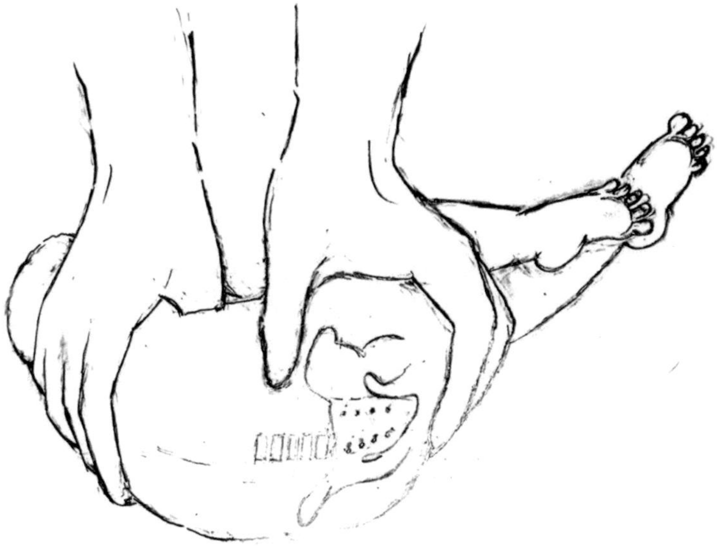

**Figure 1.** Lateral recumbent position (by Ziver Öncel).

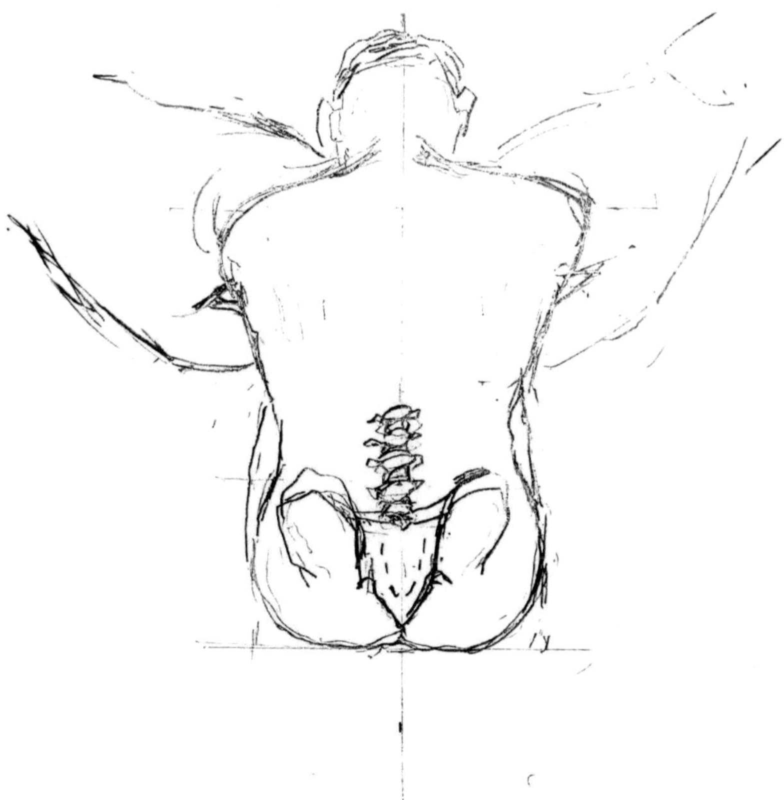

**Figure 2.** Sitting position (by Ziver Öncel).

be feasible in a still infant with the widest interspinous space (the space between the spinous processes of two adjacent vertebrae) possible. Change of position does not alter subarachnoid space width, thus does not have a role in lumbar puncture success via this mechanism [25]. Safety, as well as the ease of the LP is a very important issue in the neonatal period especially considering the vulnerability of infants hospitalized in neonatal intensive care units. In adults, studies have uniformly showed that the maximal interspinal distance can be obtained with maximal hip flexion [26, 27].

We have shown in our study, in which the infants enrolled were placed in two lateral recumbent and two upright positions (lateral recumbent without flexing the hips, lateral recumbent with maximal hip flexion, sitting without flexing the hips and sitting with maximal hip flexion), that having the patient sit with maximal hip flexion provided the largest interspinous space for the grand majority of the infants, and that the lateral recumbent position without flexing the hips has resulted in the narrowest interspinous space. Although providing significantly larger interspinous spaces, sitting positions with/without flexion have resulted in significant increases in HR with respect to lateral recumbent position without flexion. Similarly, we observed statistically significant drops in oxygen saturations between lateral recumbent and sitting with flexion, lateral recumbent with flexion and sitting without flexion, and lateral recumbent with flexion and sitting with flexion positions. No adverse hypoxic events occurred during the procedure in the entire study [28]. In adults, the position providing the significantly greatest interspinous space was obtained with the so-called "sitting, feet supported position" in which the patient touches her/his ankles while sitting [27]. This position resembles sitting with maximal hip flexion position in newborns. In a survey, most (82%) pediatric emergency attending physicians were found to opt for the lateral decubitus position [29]. Gleason et al. found that although $PO_2$ decreased and the HR increased with each position for LP, the decrease was significantly greater in the recumbent position with maximal hip flexion [30]. Cadigan et al. also found that recumbent with maximal hip flexion position provided wider interspinous spaces than did the recumbent without flexing the hips in healthy newborns in their well-child visits [24]. HR and oxygen saturation differed significantly with positioning of the infants in our study; however, this did not result in any apparent changes in clinical status. Although there were few infants weighing less than 1500 g in our study population, our results have shown that sitting-flexed position was a safe alternative to traditional-flexed recumbent position [28].

### 9.3. Landmarks

Once the patient is positioned, the most upper points of the posterior superior iliac crests are palpated. The line imaginarily drawn between these two points intersects the midline just above the fourth lumbar vertebra. The interspaces between L3-L4 and L4-L5 can then be located. Unlike children outside infancy, for whom the L2-L3 interspace may also be used, L3-L4 or L4-L5 interspace should be used for LP of neonates due to anatomical positioning explained above [7].

### 9.4. Puncture

The puncture site should be cleansed with povidone-iodine solution, which can be removed with alcohol. Sterile drapes with a hole in the center to allow for a fine exposure are placed on the procedure site. The projection of interspace on the skin may be marked by depressing a fingernail on the skin so that the puncture site can be relocated.

If not previously anesthetized with one of the topical agents mentioned above, the skin and subcutaneous tissues are infiltrated with 1% lidocaine. Local anesthesia for LP is encouraged in neonates, because it has been shown to decrease the pain response to LPs without altering their success rate [31].

Two approaches are possible for inserting the spinal needle: in the median approach, the needle is inserted through the supraspinal ligament exactly in the midline. In the lateral approach, the needle is inserted lateral to the ligament. Unlike older patients, supraspinal and interspinal ligaments are rarely calcified in children, which renders a lateral approach unnecessary; therefore the median approach is most commonly used. With both approaches, the needle may be held in one hand or with both hands. It is better if the bevel of the spinal needle is positioned horizontally in the lateral recumbent position and vertically in the sitting position, because in this way, the fibers of the dura mater, which run longitudinally down the spinal cord, are pierced parallelly, the amount of CSF leakage is minimized, and likelihood of post-LP headache is decreased [7]. The needle is then advanced cephalad toward the umbilicus or slightly caudad according to the patient's position of lateral recumbency or sitting, respectively. In the study by Bruccoleri et al., the "ideal" angle for LP as determined by ultrasonography was 50° in infants in both the lateral recumbent and sitting positions [32]. In the lateral approach, the needle should be inserted lateral to the upper border of the spinous process of L3 or L4. It should then be directed slightly medial and slightly upward (cephalad) to avoid contact with the supraspinal ligament.

It is normal that some resistance is felt during the advancement of the needle. When the ligamentum flavum is penetrated, this resistance may be lost a bit, especially in older children. There is a second resistance change when the dura is pierced. This second loss of resistance is often referred to as a "pop," which may not be evident in infants. Inserting the needle too far may result in a traumatic LP. The most effective way to avoid this problem is by inserting the needle slowly and methodically, in increments of a few millimeters at a time, and frequently checking for return of CSF. For infants under 3 months of age, the appropriate distance of insertion is approximately 1.0–1.5 cm [33]. Various studies have been carried out to determine the proper depth of needle insertion for LP. Of these studies, numerous different formulae have been developed. Taking the studies of Craig et al., Shenkman et al., Arthurs et al., and Oulego-Erroz et al., whose formulae are applicable to neonates, as examples, the ideal distances of insertion were found to be

- [0.03 × height (cm)] cm,
- [13.19 + 0.0026 × weight (g) − 0.12 × post-conceptual age in weeks] mm,
- [2 × weight (kg) + 7] mm, and
- [2.5 × weight (kg) + 6] mm, respectively [34–37].

The spinal needle should be supported with fingers during fluid collection in order to prevent dural tugging, a potential source of local pain and post-LP CSF leakage.

If no CSF is coming after the needle has been inserted into an appropriate depth, rotating the needle 90° may be of help. If this is not effective, the stylet is replaced and the needle is advanced slightly. In some cases, withdrawing the needle incrementally will result in CSF flow when the procedure is initially unsuccessful. If spinal fluid is not obtained despite such maneuvers, the procedure should be attempted again by removing the spinal needle with the stylet in place till it arrives just under the skin and redirecting it. The needle can also be withdrawn entirely and a new needle used at a different insertion site. CSF may come very slowly in dehydrated infants when LP is performed using the lateral recumbent position. Getting the patient to a sitting position may increase flow in this situation.

If bony resistance is felt when the needle is not yet advanced into deep tissues, then puncture over the spinous process is likely, and the needle should be withdrawn till it is just below the skin and redirected through the interspace. If bony resistance is felt when it went deeper, then the likely cause is inadequate spinal flexion. Directing the needle more cephalad and improving the position usually overcomes this problem [7].

### 9.5. Traumatic LP

Traumatic or unsuccessful LP a neonates is a probability in 30–50% of the time [38]. A traumatic LP may stem from improper technique. Causes include inserting the needle too far into an epidural venous plexus or through the subarachnoid space into or adjacent to the vertebral body. Nigrovic et al. found that lack of local anesthetic use and advancement of the spinal needle with the stylet in place were most prominent risk factors for a traumatic LP [39]. In the study of Glatstein et al., its incidence was independent of physician experience, sedation use or time of procedure [40]. It is also surprising for the author of these lines that the presence of a family member was not found to be associated with an increased risk of traumatic or unobtainable lumbar puncture, nor was it associated with more attempts at the procedure [41]. If blood is seen during fluid collection but the spinal needle is in proper position, the CSF often clears and the specimen does not clot. If the bloody CSF does not clear and clots form when it is collected in the test tube, then the needle should be removed and LP attempted at a different interspace with a new needle [7]. Ultrasound may minimize the number of LP attempts and decrease patient and parent anxiety by easily identifying an insertion site. It may also be useful to determine the reason for failure and the likelihood of success on continued attempts [19].

### 9.6. Measurements and tests

Measurement of CSF opening pressure is recommended during any LP when possible. The infant's struggling may be an obstacle for accurate measurement of opening pressure. The measurement is most reliable in a calm patient in the lateral recumbent position. As soon as the flow of CSF stabilizes and show pressure pulses with respiration, heartbeat, and jugular occlusion, the pressure manometer is immediately attached to the needle hub via a three-way stopcock. The pressure is measured at the highest level CSF reaches. Normal CSF pressure is 5–20 cm $H_2O$ in a child with neck and legs extended and 10–28 cm $H_2O$ with neck and legs flexed [7]. However, since an adult study reached totally opposite results, it is also possible that CSF pressure does not meaningfully decrease when the lower extremities are brought to extension from flexion in newborns. Kaiser et al. found the normal range of 0–7.6 cm $H_2O$ for newborns [42]. Of note, an estimation on CSF pressure can be made by counting the drops of CSF in a certain time. For 22-gauge, 1.5-inch needles recommended for use in the newborn period of life, the counting periods for which the number of drops counted equals the CSF pressure (in cm $H_2O$) are 21 and 20 seconds for body temperatures of <40 and ≥40°C, respectively [43].

The CSF is collected in test tubes. Approximately, 1 mL per tube is required for routine studies. The first tube specimen should be sent for Gram stain and bacterial culture, the second for quantitative glucose and protein, and the third for cell count and differential. Additional tubes may be used for viral culture, fungal culture, bacterial antigens, cell pathology, or special chemistries, if needed. After CSF collection, closing pressure may be measured as previously described. The spinal needle is removed with the stylet in place. The puncture area should be cleansed and a sterile dressing applied. It is important to remember removing the dressing after a reasonable time so that it does not become a source of infection.

## 10. Complications

LP is frequently associated with the minor complications of localized back pain without neurologic abnormalities, transient paresthesia during the procedure, and post-LP headache, all of which a newborn may fail to express in some way.

Permanent peripheral nerve damage is rare, because the spinal needle does not pierce the nerve, instead, it may move or stretch it [7].

Major complications after LP include LP-induced meningitis, epidural or subdural hematoma, acquired epidermoid tumor, damage to adjacent structures (disk herniation, retroperitoneal abscess, spinal cord hematoma), and cerebral herniation. Fortunately, these complications are quite rare. As previously mentioned, in the young infant, the lateral recumbent position for LP can cause respiratory obstruction, hypoxemia, and cardiovascular instability.

- **Infection**: LP through an area of cellulitis predictably causes meningitis. For this reason, cellulitis overlying the LP site constitutes an absolute contraindication to this procedure. An association has also been detected between performing LP in children with bacteremia and the occurrence of meningitis [44]; but in a subsequent analysis, this association was not confirmed [45]. In the absence of soft tissue infection at the puncture site, the risk of causing meningitis, epidural abscess, or osteomyelitis is rare enough to be clinically insignificant [46].

- **Spinal hematoma**: Subdural or epidural hematoma following LP has been reported with all forms of bleeding diathesis. Signs and symptoms of spinal cord compression, which develops hours to days after the procedure, include sensory deficits, paralysis, and incontinence. In most cases, LP is difficult and yields bloody fluid. In these patients, platelet counts are low or falling, and platelet transfusion has not been provided before LP [7, 47].

- **Epidermoid tumor**: Acquired epidermal spinal cord tumors can arise 1.5–23 years after LP due to implantation of epidermal material into the spinal canal during LP. The tumor manifests itself as gait disturbance, pain, and neurologic dysfunction. Experimental and clinical evidence strongly suggests that these tumors can be avoided if a spinal needle with a tight fitting stylet is used [7, 48].

- **Cerebral herniation**: This is the most feared complication of LP which may lead to sudden death. Patients with an intracranial space occupying lesions, such as abscess, hematoma, and tumor are at greatest risk. Elevated intracranial pressure manifested as focal neurologic signs seems to cause herniation much more (40%) than does elevated intracranial pressure presenting with either papilledema or abnormal manometric findings alone (5 and 1.2%, respectively) [7, 49, 50]. Risk of herniation in a newborn with an open fontanel and no focal neurologic findings is much lower. In most patients, assessment of the safety of performing LP can be made based on clinical basis. Patients who have a history of focal neurologic symptoms (e.g., focal seizures, unilateral motor paralysis), focal neurologic findings on physical examination, signs of impending herniation (posturing, Glasgow Coma Score less than 8, bilateral dilated pupils, respiratory abnormalities, abnormal tone, absent Doll eye reflex), or papilledema should not undergo LP until imaging establishes that the procedure can be safely performed [7] If meningitis or other CNS infections cannot be ruled out, the patient should receive appropriate antibiotic therapy prior to the imaging study.

## 11. Interpretation of CSF findings

Lumbar puncture is an indispensable diagnostic tool in neonatal meningitis. Direct microscopy should be performed as soon as possible, because if performed later, the erythrocytes and leukocytes likely undergo cellular lysis and escape detection. Gram- and Giemsa-stained smears of CSF should also be examined. CSF should be cultured, and if needed, sent for polymerase chain reaction. LP should ideally precede the initiation of antimicrobial therapy, but if delayed for any reason, empirical antibiotic therapy should be started immediately.

Interpretation of CSF findings is challenging in neonates, because glucose, and protein concentrations, and cell count are higher due to the high permeability of the blood-brain barrier [51] (**Table 1**).

Many experts accept 20–30/μL as the cutoff value for pleocytosis. Low CSF glucose, elevated CSF protein, and pleocytosis may indicate either bacterial or viral (especially herpes simplex virus) meningitis. One of these parameters being in the normal range cannot be accepted as

| Age | Erythrocytes (μL/L) | Leukocytes (μL/L) | Protein (mg/dL) | Glucose (mg/dL) |
|---|---|---|---|---|
| Preterm— < 7 d | 30 (0–333) | 9 (0–30) | 100 (50–290) (mostly <200) | 54 (27–99) |
| Preterm— > 7 d | 30 | 12 (2–70) | 90 (50–260) (mostly <150) | 54 (27–99) |
| Term— < 7 d | 9 (0–50) | 5 (0–21) | 60 (30–250) | 54 (27–99) |
| Term— > 7 d | <10 | 3 (0–10) | 50 (20–80) | 54 (27–99) |

d: day(s).

**Table 1.** Means and normal ranges of cerebrospinal parameters in neonates [51].

evidence against the presence of meningitis. In order to exclude meningitis, all three parameters should be normal; nevertheless, CSF findings may be completely normal in the very early course of neonatal meningitis. The most prudent approach would be to repeat LP after 24–72 hours in such boderline cases: if the infant had meningitis, pleocytosis and other abnormalities consistent with meningitis would be detected in CSF obtained in this second LP [52]. Ample number of erythrocytes in CSF may be interpreted as a clue to herpes simplex virus meningitis if the physician is sure that the LP was not traumatic. Pleocytosis is more marked in bacterial and Gram-negative meningitides than in viral and Gram-positive meningitides [6].

CSF protein concentrations higher than 100 mg/dL in term infants and 150 mg/dL in preterm neonates is consistent with bacterial meningitis and parameningeal infections, such as brain abscess, congenital infections, and intracranial hemorrhage [52]. Nigrovic et al. and Hines et al. found that CSF protein concentrations increased by approximately 1.1 and 2 mg/dL, respectively, for every 1000 CSF red blood cells [53, 54].

Glucose concentrations below 30 mg/dL in term newborns and 20 mg/dL in preterm infants are consistent with bacterial meningitis. Unlike in older children, CSF glucose to serum glucose ratio is not a reliable indicator of meningitis in the first 28 days of life, because newborns often receive intravenous glucose infusions and serum glucose concentrations can rise abruptly with stress [52]. In case of a bloody tap, assessing the CSF leucocyte count by correcting it with respect to that of the peripheral blood is not recommended in that it decreases the sensitivity and provides only a slight increase in specificity. When LP is traumatic, the wisest approach is to assume the patient is having meningitis and start empirical therapy [55]. Although no statistically significant difference in LP success rate was found between the lateral and sitting positions in infants in a randomized controlled trial, we, in order to lessen the chances of dealing with a difficult LP, favor sitting position with the legs flexed for it provides the widest interspinous spaces and is sufficiently safe [18, 28, 56].

## 12. Conclusion

Lumbar puncture of the newborn is not a smaller equivalent of the procedure performed in adults, even older children, as evidenced by its specific challenges of success and interpretation.

## Acknowledgements

The author wishes to thank Ziver Öncel (83-year-old father) and Utkan Koray Öncel (7-year-old son) for their joint work in preparation of figures.

## Conflict of interest

No potential conflicts of interest. No financial support.

## Author contribution

The author contributed as the only person to this chapter with conception and design of the manuscript, literature review and analysis, drafting and critical revision and editing, and final approval of the final version.

## Supportive foundations

None.

## Author details

Selim Öncel

Address all correspondence to: selimoncel@doctor.com

Division of Pediatric Infectious Diseases, Department of Pediatrics and Child Health, Section of Internal Medical Sciences, Kocaeli University Faculty of Medicine, Kocaeli, Turkey

## References

[1] Deisenhammer F. The history of cerebrospinal fluid. In: Deisenhammer F, Sellebjerg F, Teunissen CE, Tumani H, editors. Cerebrospinal Fluid in Clinical Neurology. Heidelberg: Springer; 2015. pp. 3-16. DOI: 10.1007/978-3-319-01225-4

[2] Frederiks JA, Koehler PJ. The first lumbar puncture. Journal of the History of the Neurosciences. 1997;**6**:147-153

[3] Moore DP, Puri BK. In: Moore DP, Puri BK, editors. Textbook of Clinical Neuropsychiatry and Behavioral Neuroscience. 3rd ed. Boca Raton, FL: CRC Press; 2012. pp. 332-334. ISBN: 13: 978-1-4441-6494-7

[4] Flidel-Rimon O, Leibovitz E, Eventov Friedman S, Juster-Reicher A, Shinwell ES. Is lumbar puncture (LP) required in every workup for suspected late-onset sepsis in neonates? Acta Paediatrica. 2011;**100**:303-304. DOI: 10.1111/j.1651-2227.2010.02012.x

[5] Malbon K, Mohan R, Nicholl R. Should a neonate with possible late onset infection always have a lumbar puncture? Archives of Disease in Childhood. 2006;**91**:75-76. DOI: 10.1136/adc.2005.087551

[6] Nizet V, Klein JO. Bacterial sepsis and meningitis. In: Wilson CB, Nizet V, Maldonado YA, Remington JS, Klein JO, editors. Remington and Klein's Infectious Diseases of the Fetus and Newborn Infant. 8th ed. Philadelphia, PA: Elsevier Saunders; 2016. pp. 217-271. DOI: 978-0323241472

[7] Cronan KM, Wiley II JF. Lumbar puncture. In: King C, Henretig FM, editors. Textbook of Pediatric Emergency Procedures. 2nd ed. Philadelphia, PA: Lippincott Williams & Wilkins; 2008. pp. 505-514. ISBN/ISSN: 9780781753869

[8] Fastle RK, Bothner J. Lumbar puncture: Indications, contraindications, technique, and complications in children. In: Post T, editor. UpToDate. Waltham, MA: UpToDate; 2017. [Accessed: June 23, 2017]

[9] Howard SC, Gajjar A, Ribeiro RC, Rivera GK, Rubnitz JE, Sandlund JT, et al. Safety of lumbar puncture for children with acute lymphoblastic leukemia and thrombocytopenia. Journal of the American Medical Association. 2000;**284**:2222-2224. DOI: jbr00199 [pii]

[10] Kneen R, Michael BD, Menson E, Mehta B, Easton A, Hemingway C, et al. Management of suspected viral encephalitis in children. Association of British Neurologists and British Paediatric Allergy, Immunology and Infection Group National Guidelines. Journal of Infection. 2012;**64**:449-477. DOI: 10.1016/j.jinf.2011.11.013

[11] Silverman R, Kwiatkowski T, Bernstein S, Sanders N, Hilgartner M, Cahill-Bordas M, et al. Safety of lumbar puncture in patients with hemophilia. Annals of Emergency Medicine. 1993;**22**:1739-1742. ISSN: 0196-0644

[12] Narchi H, Ghatasheh G, Hassani NA, Reyami LA, Khan Q. Why do some parents refuse consent for lumbar puncture on their child? A qualitative study. Hospital Pediatrics. 2012;**2**:93-98. DOI: 10.1542/hpeds.2011-0034

[13] Narchi H, Ghatasheh G, Hassani NA, Reyami LA, Khan Q. Comparison of underlying factors behind parental refusal or consent for lumbar puncture. World Journal of Pediatrics. 2013;**9**:336-341. DOI: 10.1007/s12519-013-0419-z

[14] Uysalol M, İncioğlu A, Taşdemir M, Pasli E, Olgun T. Parents' attitude and doubts about lumbar puncture. The Medical Bulletin of Sisli Etfal Hospital. 2007;**41**:23-27. ISSN: 1302-7123

[15] Tunkel AR, Hartman BJ, Kaplan SL, Kaufman BA, Roos KL, Scheld WM, et al. Practice guidelines for the management of bacterial meningitis. Clinical Infectious Diseases. 2004;**39**:1267-1284. DOI: 10.1086/425368

[16] Hasbun R, Abrahams J, Jekel J, Quagliarello VJ. Computed tomography of the head before lumbar puncture in adults with suspected meningitis. New England Journal of Medicine. 2001;**345**:1727-1733. DOI: 10.1056/NEJMoa010399

[17] Spellberg B. Is computed tomography of the head useful before lumbar puncture? Clinical Infectious Diseases. 2005;**40**:1061. DOI: 10.1086/428668

[18] Hanson AL, Ros S, Soprano J. Analysis of infant lumbar puncture success rates: Sitting flexed versus lateral flexed positions. Pediatric Emergency Care. 2014;**30**:311-314. DOI: 10.1097/PEC.0000000000000119

[19] Kim S, Adler DK. Ultrasound-assisted lumbar puncture in pediatric emergency medicine. Journal of Emergency Medicine. 2014;**47**:59-64. DOI: 10.1016/j.jemermed.2012.09.149

[20] Tumani H. Physiology and constituents of CSF. In: Cerebrospinal Fluid in Clinical Neurology. Heidelberg: Springer; 2015. pp. 25-34. DOI: 10.1007/978-3-319-01225-4

[21] Ferner H, Staubesand J, editors. Sobotta Atlas of Human Anatomy. 10th Engl. ed. Munich: Urban & Schwarzenberg; 1982. p. 88. ISBN: 3-541-72710-1

[22] Eichenfield LF, Funk A, Fallon-Friedlander S, Cunningham BB. A clinical study to evaluate the efficacy of ELA-Max (4% liposomal lidocaine) as compared with eutectic mixture of local anesthetics cream for pain reduction of venipuncture in children. Pediatrics. 2002;**109**:1093-1099. ISSN: 1098-4275

[23] Kaur G, Gupta P, Kumar A. A randomized trial of eutectic mixture of local anesthetics during lumbar puncture in newborns. Archives of Pediatrics and Adolescent Medicine. 2003;**157**:1065-1070. DOI: 10.1001/archpedi.157.11.1065

[24] Cadigan BA, Cydulka RK, Werner SL, Jones RA. Evaluating infant positioning for lumbar puncture using sonographic measurements. Academic Emergency Medicine : Official Journal of the Society for Academic Emergency Medicine. 2011;**18**:215-218. DOI: 10.1111/j.1553-2712.2010.00977.x

[25] Lo MD, Parisi MT, Brown JC, Klein EJ. Sitting or tilt position for infant lumbar puncture does not increase ultrasound measurements of lumbar subarachnoid space width. Pediatric Emergency Care. 2013;**29**:588-591. DOI: 10.1097/PEC.0b013e31828e630d

[26] Fisher A, Lupu L, Gurevitz B, Brill S, Margolin E, Hertzanu Y. Hip flexion and lumbar puncture: A radiological study. Anaesthesia. 2001;**56**:262-266. ISSN: 0003-2409

[27] Sandoval M, Shestak W, Stürmann K, Hsu C. Optimal patient position for lumbar puncture, measured by ultrasonography. Emergency Radiology. 2004;**10**:179-181. DOI: 10.1007/s10140-003-0286-3

[28] Öncel S, Günlemez A, Anik Y, Alvur M. Positioning of infants in the neonatal intensive care unit for lumbar puncture as determined by bedside ultrasonography. Archives of Disease in Childhood-Fetal and Neonatal Edition. 2013;**98**:F133-F135. DOI: 10.1136/archdischild-2011-301475

[29] Baxter AL, Welch JC, Burke BL, Isaacman DJ. Pain, position, and stylet styles: İnfant lumbar puncture practices of pediatric emergency attending physicians. Pediatric Emergency Care. 2004;**20**:816-820. ISSN: 1535-1815

[30] Gleason CA, Martin RJ, Anderson J V, Carlo WA, Sanniti KJ, Fanaroff AA. Optimal position for a spinal tap in preterm infants. Pediatrics. 1983;**71**:31-35. ISSN: 0031-4005

[31] Pinheiro JM, Furdon S, Ochoa LF. Role of local anesthesia during lumbar puncture in neonates. Pediatrics. 1993;**91**:379-382. ISSN: 0031-4005

[32] Bruccoleri RE, Chen L. Needle-entry angle for lumbar puncture in children as determined by using ultrasonography. Pediatrics. 2011;**127**:e921-e926. DOI: 10.1542/peds.2010-2511

[33] Bilić E, Bilić E, Dadić M, Boban M. Calculating lumbar puncture depth in children. Collegium Antropologicum. 2003;**27**:623-626. ISSN: 0350-6134

[34] Craig F, Stroobant J, Winrow A, Davies H. Depth of insertion of a lumbar puncture needle. Archives of Disease in Childhood. 1997;**77**:450. ISSN: 1468-2044

[35] Shenkman Z, Rathaus V, Jedeikin R, Konen O, Hoppenstein D, Snyder M, et al. The distance from the skin to the subarachnoid space can be predicted in premature and formerpremature infants. Canadian Journal of Anesthesia. 2004;**51**:160-162. DOI: 10.1007/BF03018776

[36] Arthurs OJ, Murray M, Zubier M, Tooley J, Kelsall W. Ultrasonographic determination of neonatal spinal canal depth. Archives of Disease in Childhood-Fetal and Neonatal Edition. 2008;**93**:F451-F454. DOI: 10.1136/adc.2007.129221

[37] Oulego-Erroz I, Mora-Matilla M, Alonso-Quintela P, Rodríguez-Blanco S, Mata-Zubillaga D, de Armentia SLL. Ultrasound evaluation of lumbar spine anatomy in newborn infants: İmplications for optimal performance of lumbar puncture. Journal of Pediatrics. 2014;**165**:862-865.e1. DOI: 10.1016/j.jpeds.2014.06.038

[38] Muthusami P, Robinson AJ, Shroff MM. Ultrasound guidance for difficult lumbar puncture in children: Pearls and pitfalls. Pediatric Radiology. 2017;**47**:822-830. DOI: 10.1007/s00247-017-3794-0

[39] Nigrovic LE, Kuppermann N, Neuman MI. Risk factors for traumatic or unsuccessful lumbar punctures in children. Annals of Emergency Medicine. 2007;**49**:762-771. DOI: 10.1016/j.annemergmed.2006.10.018

[40] Glatstein MM, Zucker-Toledano M, Arik A, Scolnik D, Oren A, Reif S. Incidence of traumatic lumbar puncture: Experience of a large, tertiary care pediatric hospital. Clinical Pediatrics (Philadelphia). 2011;**50**:1005-1009. DOI: 10.1177/0009922811410309

[41] Nigrovic LE, McQueen AA, Neuman MI. Lumbar puncture success rate is not influenced by family-member presence. Pediatrics. 2007;**120**:e777-e782. DOI: 10.1542/peds.2006-3442

[42] Kaiser A, Whitelaw AG. Normal cerebrospinal fluid pressure in the newborn. Neuropediatrics. 1986;**17**:100-102. DOI: 10.1055/s-2008-1052509

[43] Ellis RW, Strauss LC, Wiley JM, Killmond TM, Ellis RW. A simple method of estimating cerebrospinal fluid pressure during lumbar puncture. Pediatrics. 1992;**89**:895-897. ISSN: 0031-4005

[44] Teele DW, Dashefsky B, Rakusan T, Klein JO. Meningitis after lumbar puncture in children with bacteremia. New England Journal of Medicine. 1981;**305**:1079-1081. DOI: 10.1056/NEJM198110293051810

[45] Shapiro ED, Aaron NH, Wald ER, Chiponis D. Risk factors for development of bacterial meningitis among children with occult bacteremia. Journal of Pediatrics. 1986;**109**:15-19. ISSN: 0022-3476

[46] Eng RH, Seligman SJ. Lumbar puncture-induced meningitis. Journal of the American Medical Association. 1981;**245**:1456-1459. ISSN: 0098-7484

[47] Edelson RN, Chernik NL, Posner JB. Spinal subdural hematomas complicating lumbar puncture. Archives of Neurology. 1974;**31**:134-137. ISSN: 0003-9942

[48] Batnitzky S, Keucher TR, Mealey J, Campbell RL. Iatrogenic intraspinal epidermoid tumors. Journal of the American Medical Association. 1977;**237**:148-150. ISSN: 0098-7484

[49] Duffy GP. Lumbar puncture in the presence of raised intracranial pressure. British Medical Journal. 1969;**1**:407-409. ISSN: 0007-1447

[50] Korein J, Cravioto H, Leicach M. Reevaluation of lumbar puncture; a study of 129 patients with papilledema or intracranial hypertension. Neurology. 1959;**9**:290-297. ISSN: 0028-3878

[51] Kapetanakis, A, Hagmann, C, Rennie, J. The baby with a suspected infection. In: Rennie J, Hagmann C, Robertson N, editors. Neonatal Cerebral Investigation. Cambridge: Cambridge University Press; 2008. pp. 269-280. DOI: 10.1017/CBO9780511544750.015

[52] Edwards MS, Baker CJ. Bacterial meningitis in the neonate: Clinical features and diagnosis. In: Post TW, editor. UpToDate. Waltham, MA: UpToDate; 2017. [Accessed: June 23, 2017]

[53] Nigrovic LE, Shah SS, Neuman MI. Correction of cerebrospinal fluid protein for the presence of red blood cells in children with a traumatic lumbar puncture. Journal of Pediatrics. 2011;**159**:158-159. DOI: 10.1016/j.jpeds.2011.02.038

[54] Hines EM, Nigrovic LE, Neuman MI, Shah SS. Adjustment of cerebrospinal fluid protein for red blood cells in neonates and young infants. Journal of Hospital Medicine. 2012;**7**:325-328. DOI: 10.1002/jhm.1920

[55] Greenberg RG, Smith PB, Cotten CM, Moody MA, Clark RH, Benjamin DK, Jr. Traumatic lumbar punctures in neonates: Test performance of the cerebrospinal fluid white blood cell count. Pediatric Infectious Disease Journal. 2008;**27**:1047-1051. DOI: 10.1097/INF.0b013e31817e519b

[56] Hanson AL, Schunk JE, Corneli HM, Soprano JV. A randomized controlled trial of positioning for lumbar puncture in young infants. Pediatric Emergency Care. 2016;**32**:504-507. DOI: 10.1097/PEC.0000000000000469

Chapter 6

# Bedside Percutaneous Cholecystostomy

Michelle Maneevese, Rahul Sheth,
Syed Aziz-Ur Rahman and Joshua Kuban

Additional information is available at the end of the chapter

http://dx.doi.org/10.5772/intechopen.70500

**Abstract**

Although percutaneous cholecystostomy historically is an alternative to cholecystectomy, it is typically performed as a bridge to gallbladder removal. As a low mortality procedure, it proves itself a valuable tool in morbid patients such as the elderly and the critically ill who present with acute cholecystitis and as an alternate route for biliary access. In high-risk patients, PC can be performed at the patient's bedside in patients who are too unstable to be transported outside the ICU. PC is performed using ultrasound, CT, or fluoroscopic guidance; however, bedside PC can only be performed using ultrasound. Ultrasound is readily available and portable and allows for real-time imaging. A 2010 study performed by Donkol et al. demonstrated success rates for CT (93%), US (46%), and fluoroscopy (62%). Though US had the lowest success rate, it remains the only option for those critically ill who cannot tolerate transportation or an immediate cholecystectomy. Contraindications of PC include hemorrhage, pericholecystic abscess, gallbladder tumor, etc. Complications include bile leak, hemorrhage, sepsis, bowel perforation, etc. The gallbladder is a small organ with much pathology. Having the knowledge and skill to adequately perform this procedure is essential, especially in patients with septic shock in need of source control.

**Keywords:** cholecystostomy, percutaneous, cholecystitis, biliary, gallbladder

## 1. Introduction

Acute cholecystitis is a serious condition, which requires rapid treatment. The gold standard treatment for acute cholecystitis is surgical cholecystectomy [1–3]. In modern practice, this is most commonly performed via a laparoscopic approach [3]. Surgical resection, whether open or laparoscopic, requires general anesthesia, and therefore a certain level of patient stability. In patients who are not operative candidates, percutaneous cholecystostomy (PC) is an alternative approach.

Percutaneous cholecystostomy is a minimally invasive, image-guided intervention. The goal of PC is to quickly decompress the gallbladder to prevent gallbladder rupture and resultant peritonitis, as well as to provide infection source control. When combined with antibiotics, this is an effective way to give the body time to lessen the inflammatory response in preparation for surgery. In patients with acalculous cholecystitis, PC can obviate the need for surgery [1, 2]. Furthermore, it makes possible the ability to perform diagnostic cholangiography and access for intervention to eliminate common bile duct stones [4]. Options for image guidance include ultrasound, computed tomography, and fluoroscopy. When performed at the bedside, this procedure is done with ultrasound guidance and has the advantage of avoiding the need to transfer patients to the operating room or Interventional Radiology suite [1, 2, 6].

## 2. History

The first open cholecystostomy was performed in 1684 followed by the first open cholecystectomy in 1878 [5]. A diagnostic test in 1921 placed dye in the gallbladder by way of a cholecystostomy tube. Percutaneous cholecystostomy was first described by Radder as an alternative to immediate open or laparoscopic cholecystectomy on the basis that initial drainage of the gallbladder will result in decompression of the biliary system and subsequent resolution of gallbladder inflammation [4]. He then performed the first percutaneous cholecystostomy (PC) using ultrasound guidance in 1979 for empyema of the gallbladder [6]. Other imaging modalities including CT and fluoroscopic guidance were used starting in 1985 [17].

## 3. Indications

Acute cholecystitis is a clinical diagnosis based on history, physical exam, laboratory values and imaging. The most common cause of acute cholecystitis is cystic duct obstruction from biliary stones (calculous cholecystitis) [3]. Once the diagnosis of acute calculous cholecystitis is made, a surgical evaluation is warranted. The majority of patient will go on to surgical resection of the gallbladder. For patients with acute cholecystitis who are not surgical candidates, percutaneous cholecystostomy is indicated. The majority of PC's placed are done in the IR suite or Radiology procedure room with CT or US and Fluoroscopy image guidance [7]. Bedside cholecystostomy is indicated in patients who are too unstable to travel to IR suite for tube placement [7, 19].

There are no absolute contraindications to emergent PC placement if the procedure is lifesaving. Relative contraindications include uncorrectable coagulopathy. In some cases it may not be possible to access the gallbladder percutaneously due to intervening bowel or because of gallbladder rupture and decompression.

In addition to calculous cholecystitis, percutaneous cholecystostomy is also indicated for acalculous cholecystitis, seen often in patients in intensive care, and pregnant women where medical treatment alone is unsuccessful [7]. Acute acalculous cholecystitis is associated with a high morbidity and mortality and is thought to be a manifestation of systemic disease rather than a process confined to the gallbladder alone [8]. Because it can be difficult to recognize clinical signs of acute acalculous cholecystitis and intensive care patients are often on antibiotics and pain medication as well as parenteral nutrition (increasing their risk), percutaneous cholecystostomy can be used as diagnostic and therapeutic procedure in patients with unexplained sepsis [9]. For some, PC may be a definitive treatment for acalculous cholecystitis [1, 10].

In elderly patients with multiple comorbidities or poor general condition, percutaneous cholecystostomy can be performed safely and after removal a cholecystectomy can be performed with acceptable conversion rate [10].

In pregnant patients, acute cholecystitis is seen with lower frequency, 0.1%. The traditional management during pregnancy is conservative treatment; however, this may lead to prolonged treatment and more complications. Laparoscopic cholecystectomy is also available, though risks with anesthesia and surgery still provide significant drawbacks. For those patients with failure to respond to conservative management, percutaneous cholecystostomy is used as a temporizing measure, until the patient is able to have abdominal surgery post partum [10].

## 4. Pre-procedural evaluation

Prior to the procedure, confirm diagnosis by obtaining history and performing physical exam. All imaging available should be reviewed to confirm indication for the procedure. Cross sectional imaging should be obtained prior to bedside placement, except in emergent cases, to assess gallbladder anatomy and plan safe route to the gallbladder. Review all prior procedure notes if available.

Blood count, liver panel and coagulation profile need to be obtained and reviewed. Usually, septic patients are on broad-spectrum antibiotics. If not, broad-spectrum IV antibiotics should be given 1–4 h prior to the procedure. Some examples of acceptable antibiotics include levofloxacin 1 g, Unasyn (ampicillin plus sulbactam) 3 g IV, and ertapenum 1 g IV [11]. Analgesia and sedation should be arranged according to patient comfort and institution protocols [11].

Obtain informed consent outline the risk and benefits of the procedure. A "time out" should be performed to ensure the correct patient, procedure, and location [11].

## 5. Techniques

Percutaneous cholecystostomy may be performed using ultrasound, CT, or fluoroscopic guidance. Fluoroscopy and computed tomography generally have limited availability, increased expense, exposure to radiation, and perhaps the limiting factor, the need to transfer critically ill patients to the radiology suite. A 2010 study performed by Donkol et al. demonstrated success rates for CT (93%), US (46%), and fluoroscopy (62%). Though US had the lowest success rate, it remains the only option for those critically ill who cannot tolerate transportation outside the intensive care unit or an immediate cholecystectomy. Also, at most experienced centers that rate of procedural success with ultrasound guidance is far higher than 46%.

The patient is positioned supine with arm abducted to an arm board. Using a convex probe at frequency range 2.5–6 MHz, the gallbladder is evaluated for the best approach. Confirm liver anatomy is as expected [1, 2, 11].

In the transhepatic approach, the catheter is to pass via the bare area of the liver in order to access the gallbladder. This may be done subcostally, thought the intercostal approach is preferred to minimize tube dislodgement and kinking. When using an intercostal approach, care must be taken to avoid puncturing the diaphragm, pleura or the intercostal neurovascular bundle as it passes inferior to the rib. The transhepatic approach decreases the risk of bile leaks and colon injury, which are more common in the transperitoneal approach [1, 2, 12, 19]. Higher rates of bleeding are associated with the transhepatic approach [13].

The transperitoneal approach is a direct puncture of the gallbladder, often used in patients who have coagulopathies, which preclude the transhepatic approach. The gallbladder must be distended and in close proximity to the abdominal wall [1, 2, 12, 19]. In the author's opinion, the transhepatic, intercostal approach is the safest and preferred method.

Once a trajectory has been planned, the patient is then sterilely prepped and draped in a supine position with right arm abducted [11]. The entry site is anesthetized with 1–2% buffered lidocaine.

There are two techniques used for placement of the pigtail catheter into the gallbladder—the modified Seldinger technique, and the trocar technique.

The modified Seldinger technique consists of inserting a needle into the gallbladder under direct US guidance (**Figure 1**). The most common needle is an 18 G 10 cm hollow core needle, although smaller gauge needles can be used with 0.018 inch access systems. Aspiration of the needle should confirm bilious return. A 0.035 inch guidewire is then inserted through the needle into the gallbladder lumen. The wire should be seen looping in the gallbladder lumen with ultrasound. Use a scalpel to create a skin nick at the needle entry site and bluntly dilate this with a Kelly clamp or curved snap. The needle is removed and dilators of increasing diameters are advanced over the wire just into the gallbladder in order to dilate a tract large enough to accommodate a drain. The most common drain sizes are 8, 10 and 12 F, with larger sizes chosen for more viscous fluid. The catheter is advanced over the wire under ultrasound guidance. Once the tip enters the gallbladder, the catheter is unlocked from the inner stiffener and further advanced over the wire. The wire and stiffener are then removed, and pulling on the drain string forms

http://dx.doi.org/10.5772/intechopen.70500

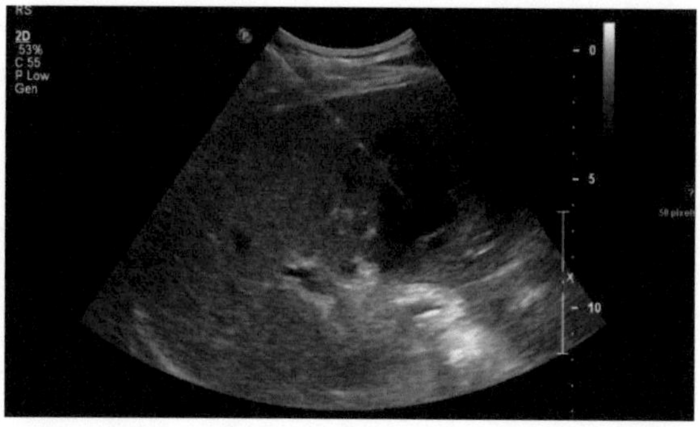

**Figure 1.** Ultrasound guided Seldinger technique with needle in the gallbladder lumen.

the catheter. This is locked into place by various mechanisms, depending on catheter manufacturer. Straight drains should be avoided, as the pigtail mechanism will help to prevent tube malposition or withdrawal. The catheter should then be aspirated to ensure bilious return. The catheter course should also be imaged with ultrasound to confirm intraluminal location of all of the sideholes. The advantage to the Seldinger technique is the use of a small needle for initial access, reducing risk of damage to surrounding structures and bleeding if the initial attempt is not successful. The biggest disadvantage to this technique is that through the multiple exchanges there is mixing of infected bilious material from the gallbladder and blood from the transhepatic tract, potentially increasing the risk for sepsis. In the case of the transperitoneal approach, this technique would allow for spillage of bilious material into the peritoneum and increase the risk of peritonitis. Furthermore, this technique requires multiple steps from initial puncture to catheter placement, making it more time consuming than the trocar technique [1, 2, 12, 19].

The second technique is the trocar technique, in which a stiff trocar needle is inserted though the drain as the inner stiffener, and they are advanced as a unit in a single pass into the gallbladder lumen under ultrasound guidance. While eliminating steps in the procedure compared with the Seldinger technique, there is a high risk of bleeding if the initial pass is not successful, as this would require multiple 8–12 F holes in the liver capsule. Damage to adjacent structures, if this does occur, would be more severe than with the Seldinger technique [1, 2, 12, 19].

After access is gained into the gallbladder (confirmed by aspiration of bile), bile is withdrawn for culture and the drain is connected to gravity drainage.

The drainage catheter is fixed to the skin with suture and a sterile dressing is applied.

Technical failure can be seen with porcelain gallbladder, thickened gallbladder wall, or small gallbladder lumen (from stones or one that is too small to accommodate a pigtail catheter) [9].

## 6. Post-procedural care

Procedure-associated morbidity can be extremely high in a critically ill patient population [14]. Although this is the best alternative to preventing/treating biliary sepsis aside from surgery, great care must be taken post procedure to avoid complications. Bed rest is needed (typically 2–4 h) with regular monitoring of vital signs and adequate pain control. The patient should be monitored for new or worsening chest /right upper quadrant pain, dyspnea, shortness of breath, and red or tarry stool. These typically occur 1–72 h after the procedure [11]. Catheter dislodgement is the most common complication and may be due to patient movement, failure to protect the catheter during transportation, or inadequate fixation of the catheter. Timely removal of the catheter after mature tract formation can decrease biliary peritonitis secondary to bile leakage [9].

The catheter should be flushed daily with 5–10 mL with sterile saline to avoid occlusion [9].

Cholangiography can be used to assess patency of the cystic duct, presence of gallstones, and catheter position days after the procedure or when the patient has stabilized [11]. Using the tube for diagnostic studies is not recommended until the patient has clinically improved from their infection.

The catheter cannot be removed for at least 6 weeks [11], unless done during a cholecystectomy. Prior to removal, two things must be established: patency of the cystic duct and maturity of the transhepatic/transperitoneal tract. These are accomplished with fluoroscopic evaluation via fistulography. This is performed with injection of contrast material to evaluate patency of the cystic and common bile ducts. To evaluate tract maturity, a guidewire is placed through the catheter and looped in the gallbladder lumen and the catheter is removed. Tract maturation is evaluated by injecting contrast through a sheath as is it withdrawn over the wire. Care must be taken to preserve wire access to the gallbladder. The tract is considered mature if there is no leakage into the peritoneal cavity. If leakage is identified, a new catheter is placed and the process repeated until maturation is confirmed [12]. If the tract is mature and the cystic duct and CBD are patent, then many operators will opt for a clamp trial of the catheter.

## 7. Outcomes

Response rates vary widely in the literature from 8 to 100% [16]. Atara et al. found the success rate to be as high as 79% in their study [4]. Patients with clinical signs and localized symptoms to the right upper quadrant are more likely to respond to PC. Patients in the intensive care unit were less likely to respond to PC [16, 20]. When the gallbladder is the only source of infection, the response is dramatic. Positive response to treatment was seen in up to 59% of critically ill patients according to a study by Boland et al. [9].

A study by Atara et al. suggests that scheduled cholecystectomy after PC may prevent biliary complications over the long term. They demonstrated a post-surgery rate of 5.6% and mortality rate was 2.8%, both significantly lower than found in the literature [4].

While recurrent rates of are low for additional episodes of acute appendicitis in the general population, the populations with high surgical mortality and morbidity have higher incidences of recurrent attacks. Removing the gallbladder ensures further episodes of biliary sepsis that can also carry similarly high mortality rates do not occur [16].

Patients who are not candidates for cholecystectomy and continue to have indwelling cholecystostomy tubes need to have routine exchanges of the catheter to prevent obstruction and/or encrustation. These are typically performed every 8–12 weeks, with shorter intervals in patients who occlude their catheters. In addition to daily normal saline flushes, Ursodiol can be given to thin bile and prevent crystal formation in patients who have issues with catheter patency.

## 8. Contraindications

There are no absolute contraindications to percutaneous cholecystostomy. Relative contraindications of PC include hemorrhage or uncorrectable bleeding diathesis, and pericholecystic abscess. A gallbladder filled with stones might prevent catheter insertion. Presence of gallbladder tumor is also a relative contraindication as tumor seeding might occur.

The presence of ascites was once thought to increase the risk of failed tract maturation; however, a 2015 study demonstrated that it is not increased when compared to patients without ascites [15].

## 9. Complications

Tube dislodgement is a frequent complication (**Figure 2**), seen as high as 80% [13]. Friedrich et al found tube dislodgement to be 59% in their study [14]. The method used for placement was proven to be unrelated to rates of dislodgement [14]. The locking loop catheters are preferred to reduce the risk of dislodgment as the catheter dislodgment tends to occur in a higher rate here

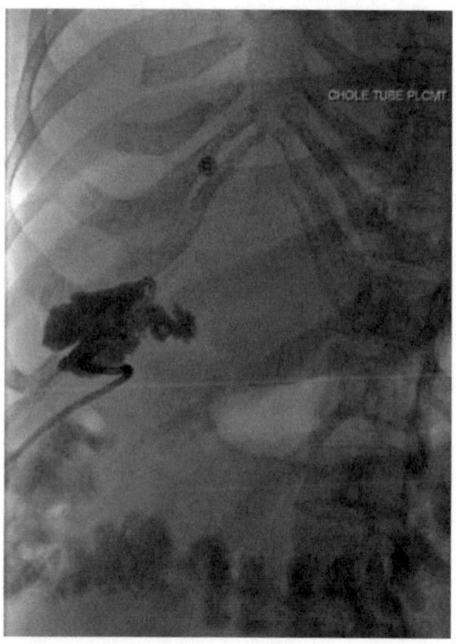


**Figure 2.** Intraoperative fluoroscopic image obtained after cholecystectomy tube placement. Contrast is seen within the gallbladder lumen after injection into the catheter.

than in other organs [4, 9]. This is mostly due to the degree of respiratory motion at this location in the abdomen and, in the author's experience, is encountered less frequently with the intercostal approach compared with the subcostal approach. Critically ill patients are also prone to altered mental status and dislodgement can be secondary to forceful removal by the patient [9].

Complications directly related to placement of a cholecystostomy tube include bile leak, cholangitis, bleeding, tube dislodgment, hematoma, biloma, seroma, pneumothorax, injury to surrounding organs including bowel perforation, abscess formation, and pain at the procedure site [14, 16].

Major complications include sepsis (3%), bile leak leading to peritonitis (4%), major bleeding (3%), and death (10%) [14].

Bradycardia and hypotension can also occur from gallbladder manipulation.

## 10. Peri-procedural imaging

The diagnosis of acute cholecystitis begins with suspicion on the basis of right upper quadrant pain and tenderness. The primary imaging modality is ultrasound, which can demonstrate stones (**Figure 3**), wall thickening, pericholecystic fluid (**Figure 4**), gallbladder distension, and

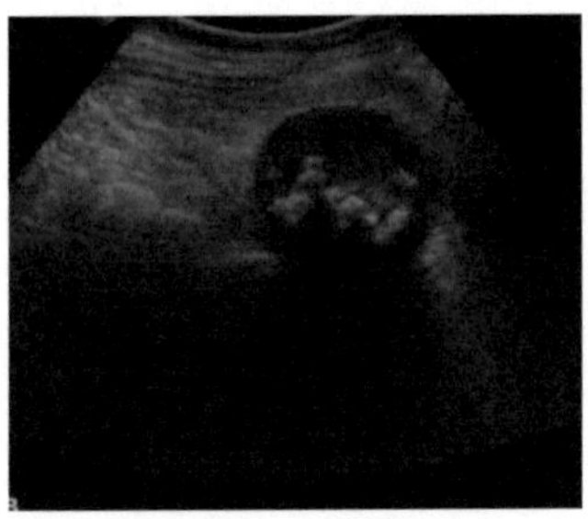

**Figure 3.** Ultrasound imaging demonstrates numerous shadowing stones within a distended gallbladder in a patient with right upper quadrant pain.

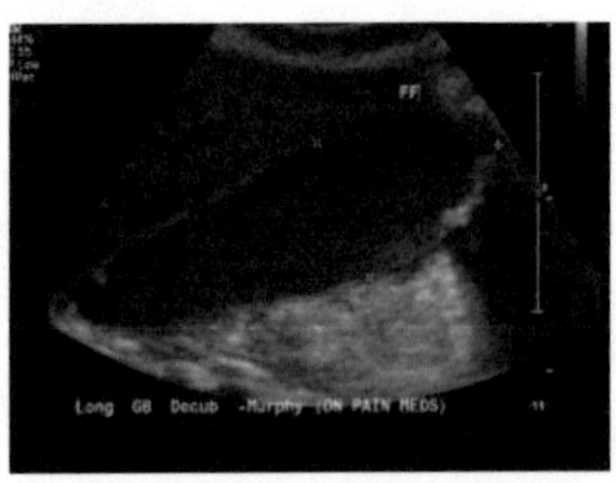


**Figure 4.** Ultrasound imaging demonstrates distended gallbladder with surrounding pericholecystic fluid in a patient with right upper quadrant pain and biliary ductal dilation.

in the absence of stones with these inflammatory findings, acalculous cholecystitis should be considered. These findings can also be seen in computed tomography (**Figure 5**). Hepatobiliary scan is used in equivocal cases (**Figure 6**) [6].

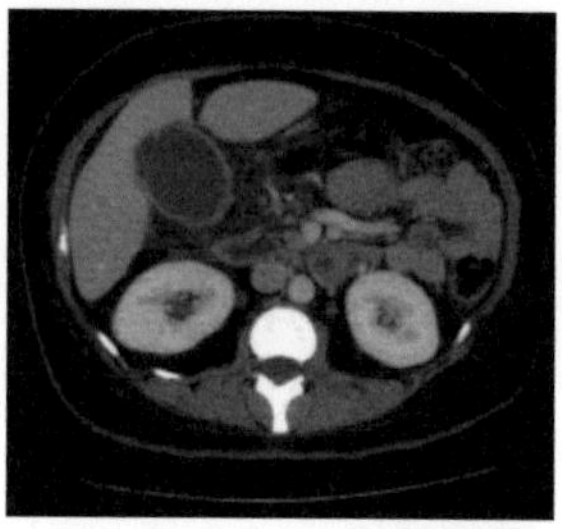

**Figure 5.** Contrast enhanced axial CT image demonstrating a distended gallbladder with wall thickening and surrounding fat stranding.

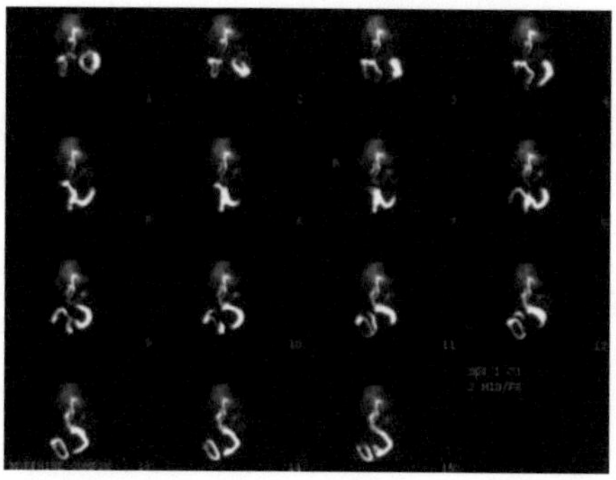

**Figure 6.** $^{99m}$Tc-HIDA scintigraphy demonstrates nonvisualization of the gallbladder after 1 h. Morphine was then administered with persistent nonvisualization.

## 11. Equipment needed

- Ultrasound machine;
- Sterile probe cover and sterile ultrasound gel;
- Sterile biopsy tray;
- Sterilizing material and applicant (chlorhexhidine stick, betadine with swabs);
- Sterile gauze;
- Sterile field cover and/or towels;
- 22 gauge needle;
- 3 10 cc syringes;

- 18 G needle;
- 1–2% buffered lidocaine;
- Kelly clamp;
- Scalpel;
- Trocar technique: 10 F locking pigtail catheter with needle trocar;
- Seldinger technique: 18 G 10–15 cm needle, 0.035′ guidewire with 3 mm j-tip, 8 and 10 F dilator, 10 F locking pigtail catheter.

## 12. Bedside set-up tips and pitfalls

As with all bedside procedures, it is vital that you have all materials needed with you. An example of tray set up is given in **Figure 7**. While many bedside procedures require tools that can be found on the ward, most of the items necessary for PC placement are only found in the IR suite or OR. Therefore, it is wise to bring a variety of tools with you, including catheters of various sizes, extra wires, dilators, and gelfoam.

Make sure to position the ultrasound screen in a convenient location that allows you to quickly look from the monitor to the access site.

Having a sterile assistant is very helpful in this procedure. While catheter exchanges over a wire are easy in the IR suite, the sterile field is more limited at the bedside and an assistant can help maintain proper sterile technique during the more challenging portions of the procedure. Have an alcohol wipe available in case the back end of the wire goes off the sterile field.

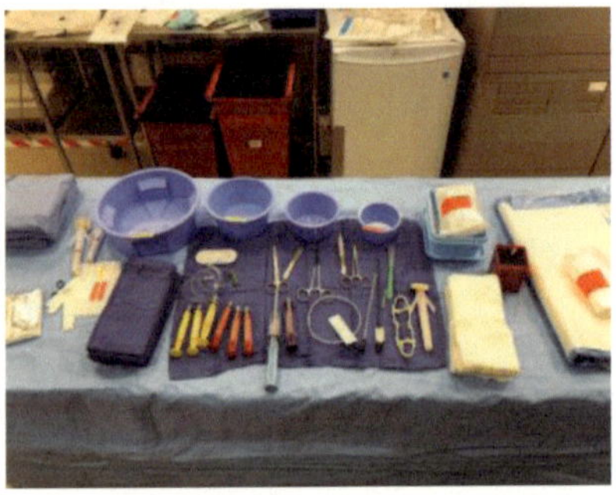

**Figure 7.** Example of tray set-up for percutaneous cholecystostomy placement.

## 13. Conclusion

The gallbladder is a small organ with much pathology. Possible treatment options for acute cholecystitis include: open versus laparoscopic cholecystectomy or open versus percutaneous cholecystostomy, sphincterostomy, or gallstone dissolution depending on the etiology. Briefly discussed was the necessity of cholecystostomy, which can be performed at bedside in critically ill patients who are not surgical candidates.

PC is a safe and effective procedure in critically ill patients in the acute phase of cholecystitis with a high technical success rate and gives added benefit of better future surgical survival and ability to remove duct stones without creating additional access [18].

Having the knowledge and skill to adequately perform this procedure is essential, especially in patients with septic shock in need of source control.

## Author details

Michelle Maneevese[1], Rahul Sheth[2], Syed Aziz-Ur Rahman[3] and Joshua Kuban[2*]

*Address all correspondence to: jdkuban@mdanderson.org

1 Department of Diagnostic and Interventional Imaging, The University of Texas at Houston, Houston, Texas, USA

2 MD Anderson Cancer Center, Houston, Texas, USA

3 Baylor College of Medicine Radiology Department, Houston, Texas, USA

## References

[1] Little MW, Briggs JH, Tapping CR, Bratby MJ, Anthony S, Phillips-Hughes J, Uberoi R. Percutaneous cholecystostomy: The radiologist's role in treating acute cholecystitis. Clinical Radiology. 2013 Jul;**68**(7):654-660. DOI: 10.1016/j.crad.2013.01.017. Epub 2013 Mar 21

[2] Blanco PA, Do Pico JJ. Ultrasound-guided percutaneous cholecystostomy in acute cholecystitis: Case vignette and review of the technique. Journal of Ultrasound. 2015;**18**(4):311-315. DOI: 10.1007/s40477-015-0173-2

[3] Indar AA, Beckingham IJ. Acute Cholecystitis. BMJ : British Medical Journal. 2002; **325**(7365):639-643. Print

[4] Atara E, Bachara GN, Berlina S, Neimana C, Bleich-Belenkya E, Litvina S, Knihznika M, Belenkya A, Ramb E. Percutaneous cholecystostomy in critically ill patients with acute cholecystitis: Complications and late outcome Units of Vascular and Interventional Radiology, Department of Diagnostic Radiology, Rabin Medical Center, Hasharon and Beilinson Hospitals, Petach Tikva, Israel Department of Surgery, Rabin Medical Center, Affiliated to Sackler Faculty of Medicine, Tel Aviv University, Tel Aviv, Israel. Clinical Radiology. 2014 Jun;**69**(6):e247-e252. DOI: 10.1016/j.crad.2014.01.012. Epub 2014 Mar 1

[5] De U. Evolution of cholecystectomy: A tribute to Carl August Langenbuch. Indian Journal of Surgery. 2004;**66**:97-100

[6] Elyaderani M, Gabriele OF. Percutaneous cholecystostomy and cholangiography in patients with obstructive jaundice. Radiology. 1979;**130**:601-602

[7] Venara A, Carretier V, Lebigot J, Lermite E. Technique and indications of percutaneous cholecystostomy in the management of cholecystitis in 2014. Journal of Visceral Surgery. 2014;**151**(6):435-439. DOI: 10.1016/j.jviscsurg.2014.06.003

[8] Laurila JJ, Ala-Kokko TI, Laurila PA, et al. Histopathology of acute acalculous cholecystitis in critically ill patients. Histopathology. 2005;**47**:485-492

[9] Boland GW, Lee MJ, Leung J, Mueller PR. Percutaneous cholecystostomy in critically ill patients: Early response and final outcome in 82 patients. American Journal of Roentgenology. 1994;**163**:339-342

[10] Boland GW, Lee MJ, Mueller PR, Dawson SL, Gaa J, Lu DS, Gazelle GS. Gallstones in critically ill patients with acute calculous cholecystitis treated by percutaneous cholecystostomy: Nonsurgical therapeutic options. American Journal of Roentgenology. 1994;**162**:1101-1103. DOI: 10.2214/ajr.162.5.8165990

[11] Kandarpa K, Machan L. Handbook of Interventional Radiologic Procedures. Lippincott Williams & Wilkins; Balitmore, Maryland. 2010. ISBN: 0781768160

[12] Akhan O, Akıncı D, Özmen MN. Percutaneous cholecystostomy. European Journal of Radiology. 2002 Sep;**43**(3):229-236; Department of Radiology, School of Medicine, Hacettepe University, Ankara, Turkey

[13] McKay A, Abulfaraj M, Lipschitz J. Short- and long-term outcomes following percutaneous cholecystostomy for acute cholecystitis in high-risk patients. Surgical Endoscopy. 2012 May;**26**(5):1343-1351. DOI: 10.1007/s00464-011-2035-0. Epub 2011 Nov 17

[14] Friedrich AU, Baratta KP; Lewis, J; Karam AR, Hudlin M, Litwin DE, Cahan MA. Cholecystostomy treatment in an ICU population: Complications and risks. Surgical Laparoscopy, Endoscopy & Percutaneous Techniques. 2016 Oct;**26**(5):410-416

[15] Duncan CT, et al. Outcomes of percutaneous cholecystostomy in the presence of ascites. Journal of Vascular and Interventional Radiology. 2016 Apr;**27**(4):562-566.e1. DOI: 10.1016/j.jvir.2015.12.004. Epub 2016 Feb 15

[16] Toh Y, Yano K, Takesue F, et al. Abdominal surgery for patients on maintenance hemodialysis. Surgery Today. 1998;**28**:268-272

[17] Yamakawa T, Fukuda N. History of surgery for cholelithiasis: From the era of cholecystostomy to laparoscopic surgery. Nihon Geka Gakkai Zasshi. 2000 Dec;**101**(12):877-881

[18] Zaroura S, Imama A, Kouniavskya G, Lina G, Zbara A, Mavora E. Percutaneous Cholecystostomy in the Management of High-risk Patients Presenting with Acute Cholecystitis: Timing and Outcome at a Single Institution. Rehovot: Department of Surgery, Kaplan Medical Center; 2017

[19] Venara A, Carretier V, Lebigot J, Lermite E, Technique and indications of percutaneous cholecystostomy in the management of cholecystitis in 2014. Journal of Visceral Surgery. 2014 Dec;**151**(6):435-439; ISSN 1878-7886

[20] Hultman SC, Herbst AC, McCall MC, Mauro AM. The efficacy of percutaneous cholecystostomy in critically ill patients. The American Surgeon. 1996;**62**:263-269

Chapter 7

# Intra-Abdominal Pressure Monitoring

Zsolt Bodnar

Additional information is available at the end of the chapter

http://dx.doi.org/10.5772/intechopen.70701

**Abstract**

Pancreatitis, inflammatory processes or retroperitoneal haemorrhage, paralytic ileus, ascites, severe visceral oedema caused by extreme fluid replacement, blunt abdominal trauma, peritonitis, or even massive transfusion can be found among the triggering factors of intra-abdominal hypertension and abdominal compartment syndrome (ACS). The only possible way of establishing the diagnosis is to measure the intra-abdominal pressure (IAP), a widespread manner of which is the measurement through the bladder. In our works, we wanted to study whether the method of continuous intra-abdominal pressure monitoring is feasible within the everyday practice of diagnosing the conditions having increased intra-abdominal pressure. The globally accepted pressure measurement carried out through a urinary catheter and its classical so-called intermittent form has been employed worldwide in the intensive care units and surgical wards. The procedure is simple, yet time consuming, and the catheter connections and disconnections are sources of infection. The measurement results provide information only on the individual pressure values of the predetermined measurement dates. In order to eliminate these weaknesses and for the safe and quick measurements, the classical technique was replaced by a completely new method: the continuous intra-abdominal pressure monitoring. In order to determine the objectivity of the continuous intra-abdominal pressure measurement technique, we carried out a validation study on surgical patients with normal and elevated intra-abdominal pressures. The pressure was determined by both methods in case of all patients. Significant difference could not be observed between the results of the intermittent and of the new technique. In this chapter, we want to discuss in detail of this validation study appointing the strong advantages of the new monitoring process. Measurement of the intra-abdominal pressure is essential in the differential diagnosis of acute abdominal pathologies. Pressure measurement through urinary catheters for the monitoring of the intra-abdominal pressure, especially its continuous variant, is an excellently applicable method. Introduction into the daily clinical routine is highly recommended.

**Keywords:** intra-abdominal pressure, intermittent intra-abdominal pressure measurement, continuous intra-abdominal pressure monitoring, intra-abdominal hypertension, abdominal compartment syndrome

# 1. Introduction

Human body is subdivided into smaller or larger units by well-defined compartments. The function of these compartments is to mechanically protect and separate from one another the organs or organ systems situated inside them. Distinctively separated spaces of our bodies are the different fascial compartments, the skull, the spinal canal, the orbit, the pericardium, and the thoracic and the abdominal cavities [1]. The elasticity of the tissues of the separating walls (bone, muscle, connective tissue) have a strong determinative effect on the tolerance for volume or pressure changes exerted on the organs, which can be found inside these compartments. Compartment syndrome in a wider sense defines those changes that occur in the given compartments due to the increased pressure (which apart from some lesser and/or greater fluctuations is constant under physiological circumstances) and to the decrease in local circulation developing in consequence of this. Detrimental effects of the increased pressure are widely known and precisely described in the medical literature [1–7]. Herniation syndromes occurring as a consequence of the increased intracranial pressure, the clinical appearance of pneumothorax and haemothorax caused by pathological accumulation of air or fluids inside the thoracic cavity, as well as the concept of pericardial tamponade are known by everybody. Although approaching these from this point of view is not routinish, yet no one questions that all the above cases represent a compartment syndrome occurring as a consequence of the increased pressure having been elevated due to certain specific reasons. Upon mentioning, associations are immediately made to fascial compartments; however, the term compartment syndrome means the clinical picture of the entirety of pathophysiological alterations developing in consequence of the increased pressure occurring within a closed space; and this is irrespective whether the separating compartment itself is formed by the skull, the thorax, the abdominal cavity, or a given fascial compartment. A common characteristic of these syndromes is the permanent and irreversible damage that may affect the organs, which can be found inside the given compartment if quick intervention cannot be provided. If vital organs are affected, these damages can be life-threatening or may even lead to death.

Abdominal compartment syndrome (ACS) was first described in relation to abdominal traumatic injuries, but its occurrence is not a bit scanty in the general surgical patient material, despite the fact that its aetiology is completely different [1, 2]. Kron [8] was the first who albeit did not use the term itself, yet described compartment syndrome in 1984. It was again Kron who routinely used abdominal pressure measurement through bladder catheterisation [8], which became widespread by 1989; however, the fundamentals of the method were described 100 years prior by Oderbrecht. Later on, several research groups developed the method [9–13]. The creation of abdominal compartment syndrome as technical term is associated with the work of Fietsam et al in 1989. The golden age of ACS has been launched by the two papers of Schein and Burch published in 1995 and 1996, respectively.

Pancreatitis, inflammatory processes or retroperitoneal bleeding, paralytic ileus, ascites, and severe visceral oedema caused by extreme fluid replenishment, blunt abdominal trauma, peritonitis, or even massive transfusion can be found among the triggering factors of ACS; i.e., all factors that may and can lead to a sudden increase in the intra-abdominal pressure

http://dx.doi.org/10.5772/intechopen.70701

(IAP, 5–10 mmHg under physiological circumstances), to conditions of intra-abdominal hypertension (IAH, IAP ≥ 12 mmHg) associated with organ or multiple organs' failure, or without intervention to abdominal compartment syndrome (IAP ≥ 20 mmHg, which is associated with the failure of vital organs) [2, 7, 11, 12]. Despite the modern and quick diagnostics and the adequate surgical interventions performed in time, the mortality of ACS is extremely high (38–71%). It affects practically all vital organ systems such as cardiovascular, respiratory, urinary and central nervous systems, as well as the parenchymatous organs.

The only possible way of establishing the diagnosis is to measure the intra-abdominal pressure. A widespread manner of measurement is the method used through the bladder [8–11]. The fundamental principle of the method is the law which says that if pressure is exerted on the surface of a compartment predominantly containing some kind of fluid, then this pressure imposed upon the practically incompressible fluid will be transmitted unaltered to each and every point of the affected compartment. Consequently, the IAP and the intravesical pressure values are strictly identical. If the bladder is filled with 50 mL of physiological saline and the previously inserted catheter is closed, then the pressure predominating the bladder will be transmitted to the catheter and become easily measurable through a sterile needle inserted into the catheter. This procedure was simplified by the working group of Sugrue [11], who placed a 'T-element' into the catheter, which rendered unnecessary the closure and insertion of it, and also significantly reducing the prevalence of infections associated with this measurement. To surmount points of weakness (laboursome, intermittent), Balogh and his working group [13] developed and validated the method of continuous intra-abdominal pressure monitoring (CIAPM). Owing to their modifications, the procedure of vesical filling, catheter closure, and needle insertion was smoothed away ('Balogh-Sugrue technique').

Treatment of ACS is nearly always surgical decompression. Within the frame of prevention or in the case of individual ACS responding well to conservative methods, non-surgical solutions may also be possible (evacuation of the intraluminar content, removal of the space occupying process, improvement of the tolerance of the abdominal wall, optimal fluid therapy, optimisation of the systemic and regional circulation) [14–16]. Success is greatly influenced by the aetiology of the given case and by the general condition of the patient. If IAP > 20 mmHg (and/or APP < 50 mmHg, where APP = abdominal perfusion pressure) and new signs of organic dysfunction are occurring, then the ACS is not responding to the conservative method, and the possibility of surgical decompression should be carefully considered.

Surgical treatment for all cases of IAH/ACS is decompression laparotomy with temporary abdominal wall closure or open abdominal treatment. Following decompression, the problem cannot be regarded as solved, and the conservative method should be carried further on (adequate medication, optimal fluid therapy) along with the constant monitoring of IAP. APP above 60 mmHg and IAP under 12 mmHg mean the solution of the IAH. If APP > 60 mmHg and IAP > 12 mmHg, then the conservative method is still well founded, but the decompression or the revision of the previous decompression is necessary in case of APP < 60 mmHg.

In the past few decades, the consensus definitions were elaborated and following several modifications were published again in 2013, the diagnostic method was brought to perfection, the therapeutic possibilities were revolutionised and developed to a high-tech level; however, the puzzling out of the pathophysiology in its entire depth and as an integer is yet to be achieved [17, 18]. It is known that the basis of the phenomenon is the co-dependent chain reaction of several physiological processes triggered by the increased intra-abdominal pressure, but the exact mechanism still remains in obscurity [14, 15].

## 2. Aims

The main goal of this chapter was the description of the advantages and disadvantages of the different techniques for monitoring the intra-abdominal pressure. In our works, we wanted to study whether the method of continuous intra-abdominal pressure measurement is feasible within the everyday practice of diagnosing the conditions having increased the intra-abdominal pressure, as well as the ACS. Our aim was not only to validate this new technique but also to bring it to perfection as well.

## 3. Comparative study of the traditional and continuous intra-abdominal pressure measurement techniques

### 3.1. Patients of the comparative study of the intra-abdominal pressure measurement techniques

To carry on the comparative study of the intermittent (traditional) and continuous intra-abdominal pressure measurement techniques, 20 patients with acute pancreatitis were involved. The selection of the patients was based on a random nature.

### 3.2. Measurement methods

The intra-abdominal pressure was measured on every patient, in every 6 hours, by both the techniques. To avoid the technical errors, all of the measurements were carried out by the same person. Patients were included into the study following the preliminary oral information and signing of the informed consent forms, for which the patients had the right and possibility of withdrawal made at any time without providing any justification.

#### *3.2.1. Traditional (intermittent) technique of intra-abdominal pressure measurement*

Prior to our study, protocolised intra-abdominal pressure measurements were never performed at our hospital. Sporadic pressure determinations were performed in one or two clinical centres; however, routine measurements defined in protocols could nowhere be mentioned. In order to carry out the initial pressure measurements, we performed intermittent measurements following the Sugrue technique [8–11]. The patients wore a simple bladder catheter (Foley balloon catheter, 16Fr-20Fr, latex or silicone). During the measurement, the urine collection bag was removed and the bladder was filled with 50 mL of physiological saline through the lumen of the catheter. In the next step, the lumen of the catheter was connected to a set designed and used for the measurement of the central venous pressure (B. BRAUN Medifix® pressure measurement scale) with or without the insertion of a T-tap. The zero point of the scaled measurement tube was designated in the medioaxillary line corresponding to the anterior superior iliac crest. After waiting for 1–2 minutes, at the end of exhalation, the value of IAP could be read off the scale in units of $cmH_2O$. The values read off should be converted to mmHg (1 mmHg = 1.36 cm $H_2O$). When the measurement was completed, the system and the bladder catheter were disconnected and the latter was connected to a urine collection bag.

*3.2.2. Continuous intra-abdominal pressure measurement*

The technique of continuous intra-abdominal pressure measurement was known from the international literature [13]. With the aid of personal consultations with the Australian working group, which elaborated the procedure (Prof. Zsolt Balogh), we perfected and further developed it, and subsequent to the elaboration of the ward protocol and of further training lectures held for the specialist healthcare workers, we—being the only such institution to do so—introduced it to the everyday routine practice. Taking into consideration the nature of the intra-abdominal pressure being oscillatory even on a daily basis, we considered the use of the continuous intra-abdominal pressure measurement technique to be essential for the everyday routine, as well as during the design of the studies. For the measurements, we used 18 Fr standard three-way bladder catheters (LubriSilTM All-Silicone Foley catheter, C.R. Bard, Inc., Covington, GA, USA). The catheter and the urine collecting bag remained connected for all the time. In order to perform the pressure measurement, the so-called flushing port of the catheter was connected to the insertion of a transducer to a 24-hour bedside monitor. The connection of the flushing port and the transducer was effectuated with a triple tap. The collapse of the bladder was prevented with physiological saline continuously perfused with the speed of 4 mL/h. The zero point for the fixation of the transducer was established in the plane determined by the axillary median line and the anterior superior iliac crest. After the system was set to zero, the measured data were continuously recorded, in which data could be easily read off from the bedside monitor. The actual IAP value appeared directly in mmHg and required no further conversion. Pressure values were read off in every hour. The IAP mean value determined on a daily basis was calculated as the average of pressure values recorded in 24 hours [3, 4].

## 4. Statistical methods

Between the two methods correlation was expressed using the Lin's concordance correlation coefficient and Bland–Altman's 95% limits of agreement, overall and also stratified for measurement time. The concordance correlation coefficient evaluates agreement on a continuous measure obtained by two different methods.

The concordance correlation coefficient combines measures of both precision and accuracy to determine how far the observed data deviate from the line of perfect concordance (i.e., the line at 45° on a square scatterplot). The coefficient increases in value as a function of:

- The nearness of the data's reduced major axis to the line of perfect concordance (the accuracy of the data).
- The tightness of the data about its reduced major axis (the precision of the data).

With all coefficient estimates exceeding 0.97 and immensely significant, the findings indicate a very high level of concordance between CIAPM and the intermittent method. Bland–Altman's 95% limits of agreement estimates are within the clinically non-significant ranges of ±2 mmHg.

## 5. Results

In order to determine the objectivity of the continuous intra-abdominal pressure measurement, we carried out measurements in patients with normal and elevated intra-abdominal pressures. Significant difference could not be observed between the results of the intermittent measurements and of the new technique. According to the statistical analysis, the concordance correlation coefficient was higher than 0.97 in all cases, which shows a strongly significant agreement between the two different techniques (**Figures 1–4**). The 95% limits of agreement of the Bland–Altman method were between the non-significant ±2 mmHg ranges (**Figures 5–8**).

According to our results, we can summarise that the continuous intra-abdominal pressure monitoring technique is a modern, safe, and accurate method for the IAP monitoring, which provides results immediately, in millimetre of mercury without the need of conversion.

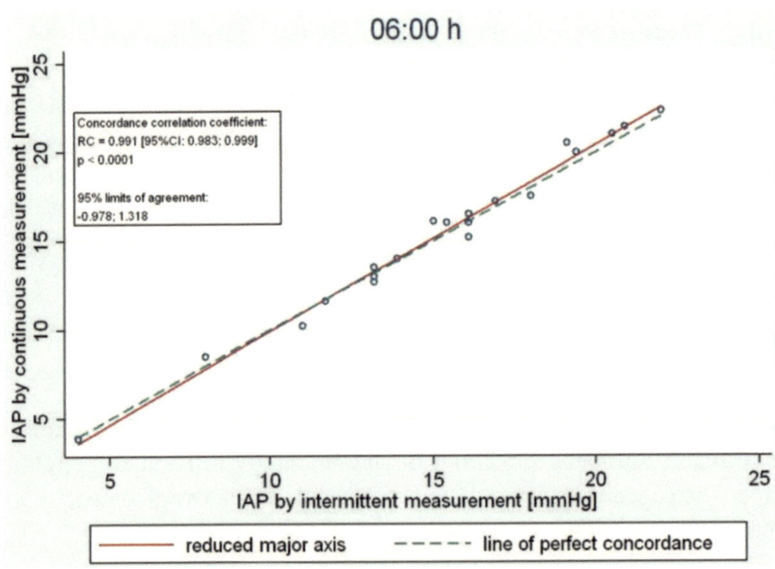


**Figure 1.** The concordance correlation coefficient was higher than 0.97 in all cases during the measurements carried out at 6.00 hour.

http://dx.doi.org/10.5772/intechopen.70701

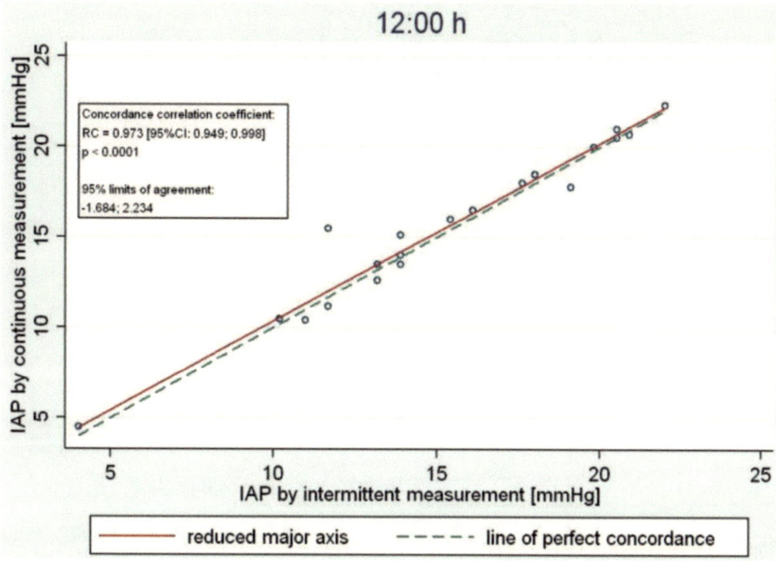


**Figure 2.** The concordance correlation coefficient was higher than 0.97 in all cases during the measurements carried out at 12.00 hour.

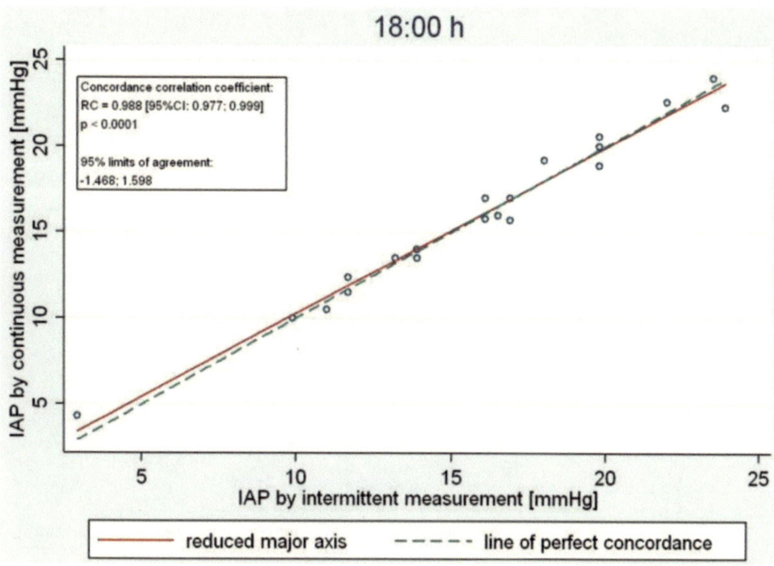


**Figure 3.** The concordance correlation coefficient was higher than 0.97 in all cases during the measurements carried out at 18.00 hour.

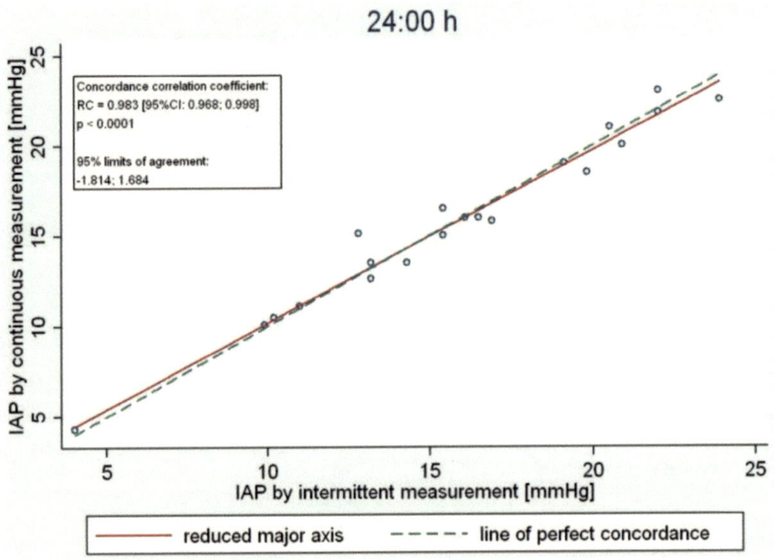


**Figure 4.** The concordance correlation coefficient was higher than 0.97 in all cases during the measurements carried out at 24.00 hour.

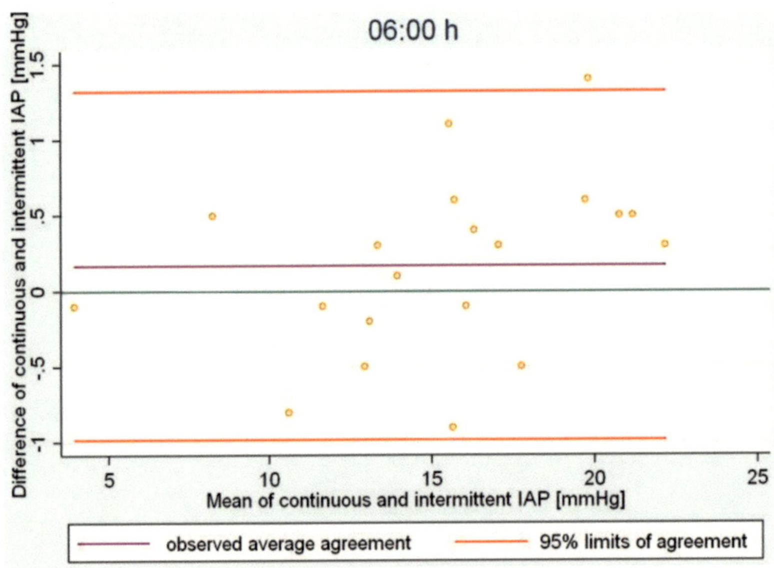


**Figure 5.** The 95% limits of agreement of the Bland–Altman method were between the non-significant ±2 mmHg ranges in all cases during the measurements carried out at 6.00 hour.

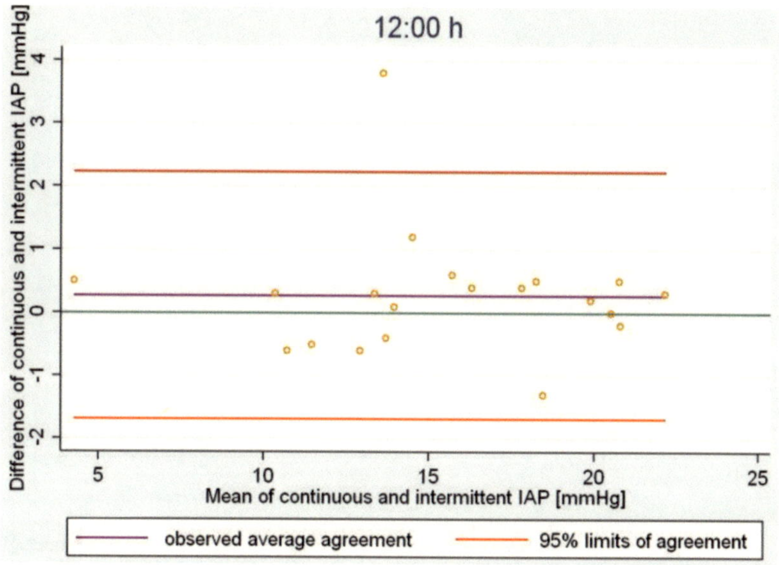


**Figure 6.** The 95% limits of agreement of the Bland–Altman method were between the non-significant ±2 mmHg ranges in all cases during the measurements carried out at 12.00 hour.

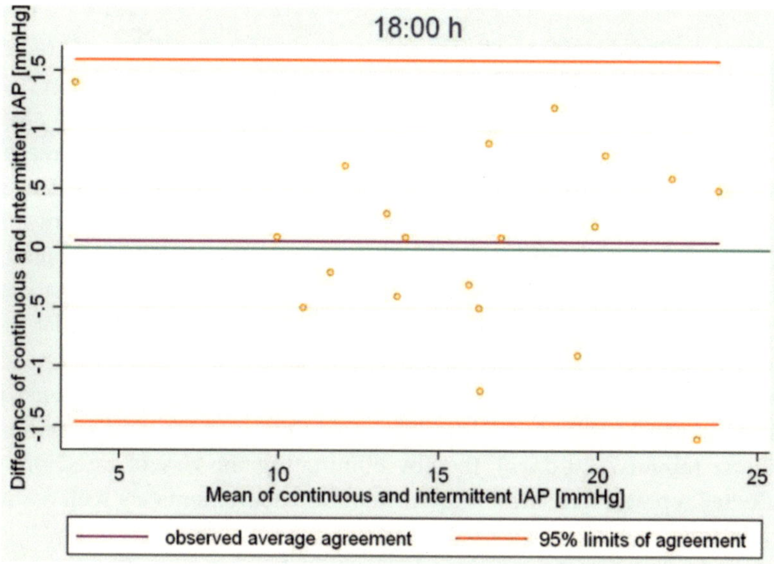


**Figure 7.** The 95% limits of agreement of the Bland–Altman method were between the non-significant ±2 mmHg ranges in all cases during the measurements carried out at 18.00 hour.

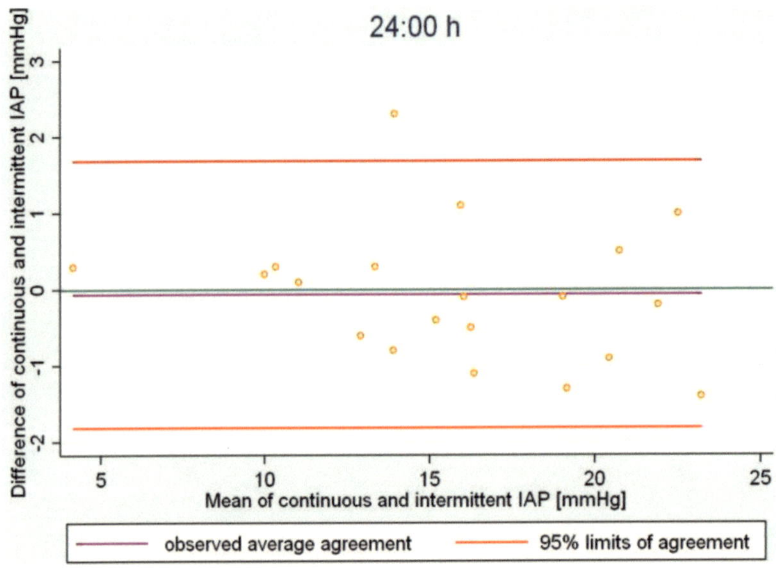


**Figure 8.** The 95% limits of agreement of the Bland–Altman method were between the non-significant ±2 mmHg ranges in all cases during the measurements carried out at 24.00 hour.

## 6. Discussion

Measurement of the intra-abdominal pressure is essential in the differentiated diagnostics of acute abdominal pathologies, in the following of surgery patients being in critical condition, in the prevention of the IAH/ACS, as well as in the monitoring of the already developed syndrome [3–5, 7–13]. The IAP (being within the normal range or increased) is never a constant value but has an oscillatory nature even less than 24 hours [12]. This nature was the main demand to develop a continuous control providing measurement method. The continuous intra-abdominal pressure monitoring technique was first published by Balogh and his working team in 2004 [13]. In order to determine the objectivity of the continuous technique, we carried out measurements in 20 patients, and we verified that the intermittent and continuous measurements are trusted methods of intra-abdominal pressure monitoring without significant differences between them. Following its first construction, the system of CIAPM can be operated without interruption until the next replacement of the bladder catheter (about 7–10 days), thereby eliminating the risk of infection originating from the catheter replacements in the intermittent measurements, as well as the need for extra work and tools.

Summing it up, the continuous intra-abdominal pressure measurement is the "gold standard" of the intra-abdominal pressure monitoring.

Pressure measurement through vesical catheters for the monitoring of the IAP, especially its continuous variant, is an excellent applicable method. Introduction into the daily clinical routine is recommended.

http://dx.doi.org/10.5772/intechopen.70701

## Author details

Zsolt Bodnar

Address all correspondence to: drbozsolt@gmail.com

Letterkenny University Hospital, Letterkenny, Ireland

## References

[1] Balogh Zs, Butcher NE. Compartment syndromes from head to toe. Critical Care Medicine. 2010;**38**:445-451

[2] Bodnár Zs, Sipka S, Hajdu Z. The abdominal compartment syndrome (ACS) in general surgery. Hepato-Gastroenterology. 2008;**55**:2033-2038

[3] Bodnár Zs, Ary F, Bulyovszky I, et al. Continuous intra-abdominal pressure measurement technique (CIAP). European Journal of Anaesthesiology. 2006;**23**(Suppl. 37):197

[4] Bodnár Zs, Sipka S, Szentkereszty Z, et al. The gold standard technique for intra-abdominal pressure monitoring in septic patients: Continuous intra-abdominal pressure monitoring (CIAPM). Inflammation Research. 2007;**56**(Suppl. 2):213-214

[5] Bodnár Zs. Intra-abdominal pressure measurement. In: Orvostechnika és monitorozás. 1st ed. Boros: Szegedi Tudományegyetem ÁOK Szeged; 2007. p. 53

[6] Kirkpatrick AW, Roberts DJ, De Waele J, et al. Intra-abdominal hypertension and the abdominal compartment syndrome: Updated consensus definitions and clinical practice guidelines from the World Society of the Abdominal Compartment Syndrome. Intensive Care Medicine. 2013;**39**(7):1190-1206

[7] Ivatury RR. Pressure, perfusion, and compartments: Challenges for the acute care surgeon. The Journal of Trauma and Acute Care Surgery. 2014;**76**(6):1341-1348

[8] Kron IL, Harman PK, Nolan SP. The measurement of intra-abdominal pressures a criterion for abdominal re-exploration. Annals of Surgery. 1984;**199**:28-30

[9] Iberti TJ, Lieber CE, Benjamin E. Determination of intra-abdominal pressure using a transurethral bladder catheter: Clinical validation of the technique. Anesthesiology. 1989;**70**:47-50

[10] Iberti TJ, Kelly KM, Gentili DR, et al. A simple technique to accurately determine intra-abdominal pressure. Critical Care Medicine. 1987;**15**:1140-1142

[11] Sugrue M. Intra-abdominal pressure. Clinical Intensive Care. 1995;**6**:76-79

[12] Malbrain MLNG. Abdominal pressure in the critically ill: Measurement and clinical relevance. Intensive Care Medicine. 1999;**25**:1453-1458

[13] Balogh Zs, Jones F, D'Amours S, et al. Continuous intra-abdominal pressure measurement technique. The American Journal of Surgery. 2004;**188**:679-684

[14] Bodnár Zs, Keresztes T, Kovács I, et al. Increased serum adenosine and interleukin 10 levels as new laboratory markers of increased intra-abdominal pressure. Langenbeck's Archives of Surgery. 2010;**395**:969-972

[15] Bodnár Zs, Szentkereszty Z, Hajdu Z, et al. Beneficial effects of theophylline infusions in surgical patients with intra-abdominal hypertension. Langenbeck's Archives of Surgery. 2011;**396**:793-800

[16] Bodnár Zs, Sipka S, Tidrenczel E, et al. Ten years experience in abdominal compartment syndrome research 2004-2014. Orvosi Hetilap. 2014;**155**(44):1761-1770

[17] Malbrain MLNG, Cheatham ML, Kirkpatrick A, et al. Results from the International Conference of experts on intra-abdominal hypertension and abdominal compartment syndrome. I. Definitions. Intensive Care Medicine. 2006;**32**:1722-1732

[18] Cheatham ML, Malbrain MLNG, Kirkpatrick A, et al. Results from the International Conference of experts on intra-abdominal hypertension and abdominal compartment syndrome. II. Recommendations. Intensive Care Medicine. 2007;**33**:951-962